LANGUAGE DISORDERS IN PRESCHOOL CHILDREN

REMEDIATION OF COMMUNICATION DISORDERS SERIES
Frederick N. Martin, Series Editor

STUTTERING
— *Edward G. Conture*

HEARING IMPAIRMENTS IN YOUNG CHILDREN
— *Arthur Boothroyd*

HARD OF HEARING CHILDREN IN REGULAR SCHOOLS
Mark Ross with Diane Brackett and Antonia Maxon

HEARING-HANDICAPPED ADULTS
— *Thomas G. Giolas*

ACQUIRED NEUROGENIC DISORDERS
— *Thomas P. Marquardt*

LANGUAGE DISORDERS IN PRESCHOOL CHILDREN
— *Patricia R. Cole*

LANGUAGE DISORDERS IN SCHOOL AGE CHILDREN
— *Mary Lovey Wood*

Forthcoming

ARTICULATION DISORDERS
— *Ronald K. Sommers*

CEREBRAL PALSY
— *James C. Hardy*

PATRICIA R. COLE

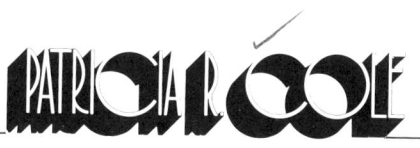

Austin Speech, Language and Hearing Center

LANGUAGE DISORDERS IN PRESCHOOL CHILDREN

Prentice-Hall, Inc., Englewood Cliffs, New Jersey 07632

Library of Congress Cataloging in Publication Data

COLE, PATRICIA R.
   Language disorders in preschool children.

   (Remediation of communication disorders)
   Bibliography: p.
   Includes index.
   1. Children—Language. 2. Speech, Disorders of.
I. Title. II. Series.
LB1139.L3C58   371.91'4   81-21000
ISBN 0-13-522862-X   AACR2

© 1982 by Prentice-Hall, Inc., Englewood Cliffs, N.J. 07632

*With Appreciation and Affection
to Jesse J. Villarreal,
a Mentor and a Friend*

*All rights reserved. No part of this book
may be reproduced in any form or
by any means without permission in writing
from the publisher.*

Printed in the United States of America

10 9 8 7 6 5 4 3 2 1

Editorial/production supervision by Virginia Cavanagh Neri
Interior design by Maureen Olsen
Cover design by Maureen Olsen
Manufacturing buyer: Edmund W. Leone

ISBN 0-13-522862-X

Prentice-Hall International, Inc., *London*
Prentice-Hall of Australia Pty. Limited, *Sydney*
Prentice-Hall of Canada, Ltd., *Toronto*
Prentice-Hall of India Private Limited, *New Delhi*
Prentice-Hall of Japan, Inc., *Tokyo*
Prentice-Hall of Southeast Asia Pte. Ltd., *Singapore*
Whitehall Books Limited, *Wellington, New Zealand*

Contents

Foreword ix

Preface xi

One

Introduction 1

THE NEED FOR LANGUAGE INTERVENTION 2
THE NATURE OF LANGUAGE INTERVENTION 4
DEFINITIONS 5
   language 5   language learning 6   language disorders 6   language intervention programs 7
SUMMARY 8

Two

The foundations for language intervention programs 9

DIMENSIONS OF LANGUAGE 10

PRECURSORS TO THE ACQUISITION OF LANGUAGE 11
   preintentional interactions 12   intentional interactions 15   prelinguistic skills: examples of disordered development 16

PRAGMATICS 18
   expressing communicative intentions 18
         expressing intentions: normal development 21
         expressing intentions: examples of disordered development 29
   language in conversation 32
         maintaining the flow of conversation 33
         maintaining the flow of conversation: normal development 33   *maintaining the flow of conversation: examples of disordered development 36*

presuppositions 38   *presuppositions: normal development 41   presuppositions: examples of disordered development 44*
deixis 46   *deixis: normal development 47   deixis: examples of disordered development 48*
summary of pragmatics 51

SEMANTICS   51
referential meanings of words 52
referential meanings: normal development 54
developmental patterns in learning word meanings 57   learning words representing hierarchical classifications 59
referential meanings: examples of disordered development 59
propositional meanings 61
propositional meanings: normal development 63
propositional meanings: examples of disordered development 66
summary of semantics 68

SYNTAX   68
learning to combine words 69
combining words: normal development 70
word order 71   prepositions 74
grammatical morphemes 75
grammatical morphemes: normal development 76
learning new sentence forms 79
new sentence forms: normal development 79
negation 79   imperatives 80   question forms 81   complex sentences 82
syntax: examples of disordered development 84
summary of syntax 85

LANGUAGE ASSESSMENT   86
the assessment process 87
information from parents 87
the observation process 91
recording speech samples 93
analyzing speech samples 94
structured assessment procedures 97

SUMMARY   98

Three

Remediation of language disorders in preschool children   100

THE STRUCTURE OF INTERVENTION EXPERIENCES   102
child-centered activities 102   group or individual scheduling 104   physical arrangements 105

INTERVENTION PLANS AND PROCEDURES   105

Contents

> children with limited interactional skills 106
>> interaction mode of behavior 108
>> demand mode of behavior 110
>> exchange mode of behavior 113
> language use 114
>> encoding intentions 114   *language to get what you want 115   language to interact with others 119   language to observe and explore the world 125   language to serve more than one purpose 127*
>> language in conversation 127   *maintaining the flow of conversation 128   presuppositions 130   questioning for clarification 136   providing clarification of intent 137   deixis 138*
> summary of intervention for language use 146
> language content 146
>> referential meanings of words 147
>> propositional meanings 150
> summary of intervention for language content 154
> language form 154
>> marking semantic relations 155
>> grammatical morphemes to modulate meaning 157
>> new sentence forms 159
> summary of intervention for language form 161

SUMMARY   162

References 165

Index 175

Foreword

With the information explosion of recent years there has been a proliferation of knowledge in the areas of scientific and social inquiry. The speciality of communicative disorders has been no exception. While two decades ago a single textbook or "handbook" might have sufficed to provide the aspiring or practicing clinician with enlightenment on an array of communication handicaps, this is no longer possible—hence the decision to prepare a series of single-author texts.

As the title implies, the emphasis of this series, *Remediation of Communication Disorders,* is on therapy and treatment. The authors of each book were asked to provide information relative to anatomical and physiological aspects of each disorder, as well as pathology, etiology and diagnosis to the extent that an understanding of these factors bears on management procedures. In such relatively short books this was quite a challenge: to offer guidance without writing a "cookbook"; to be selective without being parochial; to offer theory without losing sight of practice. To this challenge the series' authors have risen magnificently.

For more than fifteen years Patricia Cole's primary clinical activities have been with young children who have language disorders. Dr. Cole has developed a strong interest in the theoretical bases for language learning which leads to direct intervention with children. Her private practice has been devoted to an understanding of the needs of learning disabled children in all facets of their lives, while she has engaged in active participation in the political and educational arenas as an advocate for handicapped persons. Dr. Cole's skills and dedication are revealed in the pages of this book which serves both the academician and practicing clinician extremely well.

FREDERICK N. MARTIN
Series Editor

Preface

In fifteen years of professional practice as a speech-language pathologist, my experiences in working with children with language disorders have provided continuous rewards, frustrations, and challenges. The greatest sense of pride and pleasure comes when children who have gone through language remediation emerge with a grasp of language that supports their doing whatever they choose to do, within the limitations imposed by their basic potential for learning or by irreversible handicapping conditions. When this happens, it seems as though a child has gained access to a basic human right which most people have never been denied. Equally as rewarding is the discovery or recognition of some new bit of information about what children learn when they learn language, and how or when or why normal or language-disordered children learn as they do. Finding a missing part and recognizing where it fits into the language system provides a sense of excitement and relief. At the same time, it reveals new questions and alters the focus of old ones. Consideration of the complexities and the capabilities of language use is both a challenge to and a responsibility of persons who plan and implement language remediation programs.

The challenges and frustrations associated with working with language-disordered children accompany the rewards. The only thing more baffling to a language clinician than the child who does not learn language through the procedures employed in intervention programs is the child who achieves all the specific goals of intervention and seemingly should, or even does, "graduate" from the program, yet still does not use language normally. Having maintained contact with many language-disordered children from a preschool age through their elementary or teenage years, I have found that an alarming number continue to experience difficulties in using the language system effectively. Too many continue to be extremely literal in their interpretation of what they hear or read and to be inappropriately blunt, inflexible, or vague in their phrasing of what they say. Some sound "programmed" when they speak (and their speaking patterns often have an all-too-familiar cadence to those of us who taught them, through drill, to say certain linguistic forms). Many of these children have been dismissed from remediation programs, either because we thought we had taught them sufficiently and successfully or because we did not know what else to do with them. Some withdrew because they or their parents no longer felt that special programs were necessary or beneficial or because they moved to areas where such assistance was not available. For whatever reason, they are there, still burdened by a defective language system. They represent our frustrations and our challenges.

Since the mid-1970s, research in normal language learning has provided new information which adds an important dimension to our efforts to assist children who are not learning language normally. Our better understanding of language use—of the pragmatics of language—is suggesting different goals and approaches for language intervention. The evidence is building to support the notion that children learn language form and content as mastery of these aspects facilitates their use of language to accomplish certain purposes. Additionally, we are recognizing that learning language includes learning to select the linguistic structures that are appropriate in the context of their use. Our expanding information about the pragmatics of language indicates that language use should be the core around which language intervention goals and strategies are developed. Rather than beginning with goals for teaching language-disordered children linguistic structures, we should emphasize their learning to use language meaningfully and effectively and teach content and form as it relates to language use. This emphasis should reduce the likelihood that language-disordered children will "graduate" from intervention programs yet be unable to apply, generalize, and expand beyond what they learned in remediation.

Bases and procedures for language intervention programs for preschool children with language disorders are the topics discussed in this book. The rather extended discussion of normal language learning in Chapter Two reflects my contention that persons responsible for language remediation programs must understand normal development in order to understand disordered development. Additionally, readers need to recognize the theoretical bases for the intervention plans and procedures discussed in Chapter Three if they are to evaluate the efficacy of the recommendations for remediation and to apply and expand the procedures that are proposed. Understanding the theory that underlies the remediation proposals will allow readers to identify those aspects that do not coincide with their biases, to integrate new information into the plans and procedures for remediation, and to come up with specific strategies beyond those mentioned in Chapter Three.

Chapter Two begins with a discussion of the development of prelinguistic behaviors that are precursors to language learning. That discussion is included because for some language-disordered children, intervention should focus on the acquisition of preverbal communication skills in order to prepare the child for learning language. The bulk of the second chapter addresses children's learning of language use, content, and form. For each of these dimensions of language, patterns of normal development are discussed and examples of behaviors indicating abnormal development are given.

The heavy emphasis on language use in Chapters Two and Three is not unintentional. I have emphasized this dimension of language for several reasons. First, learning to use language effectively is both the primary motivation and the ultimate reason for learning language. Second, especially for young children, language content and form are learned within the contexts of language use. Therefore teaching language-disordered children to use language effectively provides the context for teaching language content and form. Third, language learned in the remediation situation is of value only if it is put to use outside of that setting. Therefore understanding how children use language in their natural environments and incorporating this knowledge in language-teaching procedures should increase the probability that they will apply what they learn when they go into other situations. Fourth, most currently available plans and procedures for language remediation emphasizes teaching language content and form, giving little attention to language use. Readers have ready access to other sources which specifically (and sometimes narrowly) suggest plans for addressing disorders of content and form. Within the discussion, readers will be referred to sources that emphasize these two dimensions of language.

Chapter Two concludes with a very brief discussion of language assessment. This discussion points out some of the considerations that I find important in assessing language. Readers will be referred to sources that address in more detail the assessment aspect of language remediation.

Chapter Three addresses content and strategies for remediation of language disorders in young children. Intervention procedures are discussed for deficits at different stages and for different components of language, with primary emphasis on teaching young children to use language effectively. The intervention suggestions are founded on information about language learning discussed in Chapter Two. While the focus is on management of preschool children, many of the suggestions are appropriate for school-age children who may not have acquired those language skills that normally are learned in the preschool years. Additionally, many of the principles that underlie the suggestions for teaching language in the early stages also apply to teaching language skills normally not acquired until school-age.

Whether or not readers concur with the conclusions about language learning and intervention proposed in this book, it is hoped that the discussion evokes or reinforces in readers a determination to plan and carry out intervention programs founded on a well-thought-out philosophy of language and language disorders. Such determination should cause those responsible for language intervention programs to approach the remediation process systematically and to take advantage of the growing body of information about language, language learning, and language disorders. Children with disordered language will benefit from such an approach to remediation.

I want to express my appreciation to many people who guided and supported the writing of this book: Alice Richardson and Mary Lovey Wood, who provided many suggestions for alterations of various drafts along the way; Martha McGlothlin, who proofread the manuscript and, as my co-worker, provided a great deal of assistance and support; Fred Martin, who, as editor of this series, was patient and encouraging throughout the writing; and Norma Rees, who, at the publisher's request, reviewed the book and supplied detailed and insightful comments and suggestions which were most helpful. To the parents of many language-disordered children with whom I work, I owe extreme gratitude. Their observations of their children and their questions and comments have guided me to recognize important details about language disorders and about intervention goals and strategies. A special thanks goes to my family and friends for providing the interest, support, humor, and perspective that were necessary during the preparation of this book.

PATRICIA R. COLE

ONE

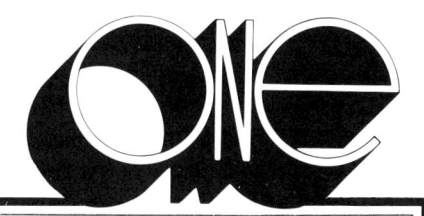

- THE NEED FOR LANGUAGE INTERVENTION
- THE NATURE OF LANGUAGE INTERVENTION
- DEFINITIONS
    - language
    - language learning
    - language disorders
    - language intervention programs
- SUMMARY

Introduction

One

Children learn language because it facilitates their communication with persons in their environment. Language provides a mechanism by which they establish interpersonal relationships, regulate the behavior of others, satisfy material needs or desires, explore and organize their environment, and exchange messages and information with other people (Halliday 1973). If language is to serve an appropriate communicative function, children must learn to use the conventional linguistic code of their community as a means of sharing ideas, experiences, information, needs, and feelings. Learning language means learning to use linguistic structures which, in the contexts of their occurrence, both represent desired content and bring about the intended results.

Most children move through common stages of language acquisition at a fairly predictable rate and with no need for special instruction. However, some children fail to learn language at the accepted rate or in the predicted manner. They do not progress normally in learning to interpret what others say or in learning to use linguistic forms for communicating appropriately with other people. Compared with their age peers, their effectiveness in using language is restricted. Children who do not learn language normally often are entered into remediation programs and receive special instruction from speech-language pathologists or other appropriately trained professionals.

○ THE NEED FOR LANGUAGE INTERVENTION

Why are special programs needed for children with abnormal language? Consideration of this question is important to persons responsible for remediation, since it will influence the nature of the program they institute; to parents, because it will assist them in deciding whether to enter their child into a special program; to legislators, agency directors, or other persons responsible for establishing and funding programs; and to education, health care and other professionals who must decide whether to refer children to specialists in child language and its disorders for possible admission into remediation programs. Recognition of the role of language in the life of young children illuminates the importance of intervention programs for those who are not learning language normally.

Language influences cognitive growth. Concepts are formed through categorization of stimuli according to sets of similar features. Bowerman explains:

> Things that are not identical but which are treated as if they were equivalent, at least under certain circumstances, constitute a *category,* or, alternatively, a concept or class. (1976, p. 105)

Prelinguistically, children develop concepts as a result of their perceptual, sensorimotor, and social experiences. That conceptual development prior to the acquisition of language influences language learning is well documented (Sinclair-de Swart 1973; Brown 1973; Slobin 1973; Nelson 1973). The influence of language on cognitive development is less frequently emphasized but equally as important.

As children learn language, preverbal cognitive categories are reorganized and redefined so that concepts relevant in the native language are developed. Children must recognize the boundaries for concepts represented linguistically if they are to use language successfully for exchanging messages. In the process of learning language, their attention is directed toward organizing objects, events, and experiences into classes that have linguistic relevance. Schlesinger (1974) states, "... by learning the meanings of words the child learns how to categorize the entities these words stand for" (p. 145). In other words, children's learning of their native language is instrumental in shaping their cognitive development.

Children use language to control other people. From the earliest appearance of speech, children demand or request actions of others, direct what other people are to do, and issue threats, warnings, or promises for the purpose of controlling someone else's behavior. They learn to alter what they say and how they say things to influence another person's decisions and responses. Children who do not learn language normally may not be able to use language to control what other people do.

Children use language to facilitate their interactions with others. Halliday (1973, 1977) points out that by two years of age, children have begun using verbalizations to establish and maintain relationships with other people. He states:

> Even the closest of the child's personal relationships, that with his mother, is partly and, in time, largely mediated through language; his interaction with other people, adults and children, is very obviously maintained linguistically. (Halliday 1973, p. 5)

Children use language to exchange information with other people. While the use of language for this purpose is not predominant in the initial stages of language learning, older children and adults share their knowledge and understandings of the world through verbal exchanges. By talking with someone else, a child can learn from the experiences of another person.

Language assists children in establishing their self-identity. Rees (1973) explains that through language, children express their awareness of themselves separate from other people and objects. The linguistic system serves as a mechanism by which they can reveal their feelings, interests, attitudes, and attributes, thereby defining their distinct identity for themselves and for others.

The acquisition of spoken language is an important prerequisite for success in learning written language. Richardson (1979) reports, "We know that one of the earliest indications of possible school difficulty is delay in the acquisition and use of language" (p. 76). Pick emphasizes the relationship between learning to read and spoken language abilities:

> ... all the models of reading that have been proposed to date acknowledge explicitly that the language that children have acquired prior to formally learning to read is an important basis for what it is that they learn when they learn to read. (1978, p. 107)

Similarly, Bangs states:

> Reading is the ability to gain meaning from a structured system of written signs which are used to represent oral language. The oral symbol, then, becomes the referent for its written counterpart. (1968, p. 16)

Aram and Nation (1980) found that children identified as having deficient language as preschoolers were likely to have oral and written language problems when they reached school age. Their findings indicate that preschool children with language disorders often do not "outgrow" their language deficiencies.

This brief overview of some of the roles which language plays indicates that children whose language is deficient may be penalized in cognitive development, in social and interpersonal growth, in the acquisition of knowledge, in establishing self-identity, and in academic achievement. Special intervention programs which facilitate a child's acquisition of language should reduce and possibly prevent subsequent problems in a variety of areas of behavior and learning considered important in our society.

○ THE NATURE OF LANGUAGE INTERVENTION

Language remediation programs are intended to assist children in acquiring language skills which are as nearly normal as possible. Special programs are instituted with the expectation that those who are not learning their native language normally will, under proper circumstances, learn to use the linguistic system more effectively and acceptably. The setting for intervention may vary according to the needs of a child, the structure of the service delivery agency, and the philosophy of the service provider. Regardless of the manner of service delivery, the primary goal of intervention is for the child to become a more competent language user.

Persons responsible for intervention programs make decisions about what the child should learn at given times and how to facilitate the desired learning. These decisions are reflected in the goals and procedures for the remediation programs. Remediation specialists' selection of content and strategies should be based on their persuasions about language, factors that contribute to normal and abnormal language learning and use, problems that result from abnormal language, and the desired outcome of the remediation efforts. In other words, persons responsible for intervention should select and sequence remediation strategies on the basis of their philosophy of what is to be learned, the order in which it should be learned, the necessary prerequisites for learning it, and procedures that will facilitate the desired learning. Unless service providers develop remediation programs from a theoretical framework, approaches are likely to be disjointed and unlikely to result in maximally positive changes in the child's communicative competence.

○ DEFINITIONS

The content of this book reflects the author's philosophy of language, language learning, language disorders, and language intervention goals and procedures. The readers' interpretations of the meanings of these terms will influence their understanding and evaluation of the statements made throughout the discussion. The following explanations are given so that readers will approach the remainder of the book with an awareness of the author's intended meanings. Later sections include a discussion of the bases for these definitions and, hopefully, demonstrate the interrelationships among the concepts underlying them.

language

The term *language* refers to a system of verbal symbols used by humans to codify ideas and experiences most often for the purpose of communicating with other people. The major components of the system and their interrelatedness are recognized in the following statement by Bloom and Lahey:

> Language consists of some aspect of *content* or meaning that is coded or represented by linguistic *form* for some purpose or *use* in a particular context. (1978, p. 11)

In the present discussion, the components defined by Bloom and Lahey provide a framework for considering language development and remediation. The dimension of content will be referred to as the *semantic* component of language. Linguistic form or structure will be considered as the *syntactic* component. Language use and function will be referred to as the *pragmatic* dimension of language.

Language is a part of a broader communication system which includes nonverbal as well as verbal behaviors. While the primary emphasis in this book is placed on the use of spoken language, it is necessary to relate verbal to certain nonverbal behaviors and conditions in order to consider many of the factors that influence language and that are essential to communication.

language learning

In acquiring their native language, children learn to use linguistic forms in appropriate contexts to represent their ideas and feelings about the world and to achieve desired results. Lahey and Bloom (1977) state, "Language learning involves inducing the relationships among ideas of the world, linguistic forms, and communication" (p. 340). Certain language forms are learned because they express specific content (Bowerman 1973a, b; Brown 1973) or accomplish certain purposes (Halliday 1973, 1977). Other linguistic structures seem to be purely formal and are learned through general inductive strategies that allow children to recognize regularities in linguistic input and to learn to employ such structures in a conventional manner (Dore 1975).

Children learn language as a part of a communication system whose roots are found in cognitive development (Piaget and Inhelder 1969; Brown 1973; Slobin 1973) and social experiences (Bruner 1975; Lewis 1978; Snow 1978). Through interactions with objects and people, they draw conclusions about entities and occurrences, about social and interpersonal relationships, and about possibilities for representing objects and events as well as feelings, desires, and intentions. Adults contribute in important ways to children's acquisition of language. Largely through interactions first with their primary caregivers and later with other people, young children learn to relate meaningfully with others and to recognize the roles language can have in their lives. Adults provide models of the conventional linguistic system within a social environment. To understand language learning, one must consider the social context in which language is learned.

Throughout this book, the terms *language learning, language acquisition,* and *language development* will be used synonymously.

language disorders

Children are considered to have a language disorder when, by comparison to their age peers, they have not learned to use language effectively or acceptably for communicating with other people. Language may be viewed as disordered because of a child's inability to exchange messages accurately through verbalizations or because the child's style or form of message transmission does not meet the standards of acceptability within his or her linguistic community (Siegel and Spradlin 1978).

Children with language disorders are not a homogeneous group. They may demonstrate deficiencies in any of the various aspects of meaning, structure, or use of language. Because these dimensions are interrelated, many children with significant deficits in one dimension will have some degree of disorder in others.

A wide range of terminology is used to refer to children who are not learning language normally. The terms *disordered language, deviant language,* and *deficient language* will be used to refer to language which is inadequate in meaning, structure, and/or use.

language intervention programs

Systematic arrangements of circumstances designed to assist children with disordered language in learning to use their native language for more effective and acceptable communication are referred to as *language remediation* or *language intervention* programs. Since language learning is dependent on the acquisition of prelinguistic communicative skills, remediation programs may appropriately address prelinguistic as well as linguistic development. Because language is learned and used in a social context that includes linguistic and nonlinguistic information, language intervention programs should integrate the verbal with the nonverbal environment.

Language intervention strategies should "provide a model of the language world to the child and should present him or her with opportunities to participate fully in using that model" (Holland 1975, p. 519). Regardless of the setting of the remediation program, activities should be organized so that the child is an active participant and so that the language learned is useful in experiences the child will encounter in outside settings. Activities should be selected and presented in a manner that leads the child to recognize that language is an effective tool for communicating with other people.

Information about normal language development provides a sound basis for selecting content and strategies for remediation programs for most preschool children with disordered language. It suggests a logical basis for sequencing of content, provides information about the interrelationships among the components of language in the developmental process, and suggests strategies which seem to enhance or inhibit language learning. Use of normal developmental data does not imply that programs for all language-disordered children should have the same emphasis. Obviously, the nature of the child's language deficits will determine which of the dimensions of language should be the focus of remediation procedures as well as the level of language complexity that should be emphasized.

SUMMARY

Children learn language because it assists them in communicating with other people and in organizing and learning about their surroundings. Those who fail to learn language normally may be classified as language-disordered. Their language may be defective in use, content, and/or form. Children with language disorders may be affected adversely in cognitive development, in social and emotional adjustment, and in academic achievement. They are entered into language intervention programs with the expectation that, under appropriate circumstances, they will learn to use the linguistic system more normally.

Persons responsible for language intervention programs must set goals and select strategies which they believe will be maximally effective for teaching the language-disordered child. Their choices are based on their knowledge and philosophy of language, language disorders, and language remediation. The focus of this book reflects the author's contentions that (1) plans for intervention with young language-disordered children should be developed and implemented on the basis of what is known about normal language development, and (2) language use should be the central point around which remediation programs are built. The emphasis on the pragmatics of language in the discussions of normal development and of remediation procedures is intentional. This emphasis was chosen for two primary reasons. First, effective language use is the ultimate goal of any intervention efforts and should be an integral part of remediation programs. Second, language use is not the focus of most discussions of or programs for management of language-disordered children. Suggestions for teaching language content and form, which certainly are important aspects of language remediation, are plentiful in other sources available to readers.

TWO

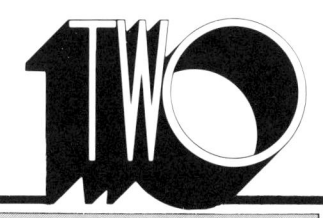

- DIMENSIONS OF LANGUAGE
- PRECURSORS TO THE ACQUISITION OF LANGUAGE
  - preintentional interactions
  - intentional interactions
  - prelinguistic skills: examples of disordered development.
- PRAGMATICS
  - expressing communicative intentions
  - language in conversation
  - summary of pragmatics
- SEMANTICS
  - referential meanings of words
  - propositional meanings
  - summary of semantics
- SYNTAX
  - learning to combine words
  - grammatical morphemes
  - learning new sentence forms
  - syntax: examples of disordered development
  - summary of syntax
- LANGUAGE ASSESSMENT
  - the assessment process
- SUMMARY

The foundations for language intervention programs

TWO

Persons responsible for planning and implementing language intervention programs establish goals and select strategies they believe will bring about improved language skills in children with language disorders. Waryas and Stremel-Campbell (1978) point out the need for consideration of the theoretical bases for remediation procedures:

> It is important for the applied language practitioner to recognize that all language intervention procedures partake of theoretical biases, either explicitly or implicitly. In other words, when a decision is made to adopt one training procedure, the practitioner is also making a judgment about its theoretical principles. (p. 147)

The information in this chapter represents the theoretical bases from which the intervention plans and procedures in Chapter Three were developed. The discussion begins with a brief explanation of the dimensions of language that are the focus of attention in the subsequent sections of Chapter Two and in Chapter Three. To recognize the continuity in the development of preverbal to verbal communication behaviors, highlights of the acquisition of behaviors that are the precursors to language are presented as a prelude to consideration of normal language learning. The discussion of normal development addresses young children's learning of language use, content, and form. For each of these dimensions, information about normal acquisition and examples of disordered development are given. Following the consideration of normal acquisition, procedures for assessing child language are discussed briefly.

○ DIMENSIONS OF LANGUAGE

Language is learned in a social context as a part of a system of communicative acts. Certain preintentional caregiver-infant routines provide a model for interaction into which intentional communicative behaviors later are incorporated. Prelinguistically, infants learn to use persons and objects in a manipulative fashion to achieve desired items or assistance, and they subsequently evidence an intent to communicate their demands, wishes, and needs to another person through their actions. Infants' uses of vocalizations and gestures for the purpose of signaling their intents to someone else are their first deliberate communicative acts. These acts may be devoid of propositional content, but interpreted within the context of their occurrence, they generally are effective in indicating what the child intends to accomplish. In other words, the meanings of early communicative acts are the child's intended effects in performing them. These systematic prelinguistic acts serve a communicative function in the context in which they are used. They have *pragmatic* meanings later expressed and expanded through language.

After learning to use nonverbal acts to bring about certain results, children learn words and word combinations to represent events, entities, ideas, feelings, and intentions. When children learn linguistic forms to stand for actions, items, and other kinds of meanings, their language has referential and propositional content. They have added a *semantic* component to their language system.

At first, children use single-word utterances, generally in combination with nonverbal contextual clues, to communicate meanings to other people. When they learn to combine words to signal meanings beyond those represented by single words, they have added a *syntactic* component to their language system. The syntactic aspect of language grows to include a variety of linguistic forms to mark different meanings and intentions.

The pragmatic, semantic, and syntactic dimensions of language can be described separately, although their learning and application are interrelated. An understanding of these dimensions of language and their acquisition is important to understanding normal and abnormal language and therefore to planning and carrying out language intervention programs.

○ PRECURSORS TO THE ACQUISITION OF LANGUAGE

From the time of birth, interpersonal interactions provide the social context in which children learn to communicate. Bruner (1978) states that "many of the conventions that underlie the use of language are learned prior to the onset of articulate phonetic speech" (p. 22). Interaction routines that become systematized prelinguistically provide a framework for children's subsequent learning of the linguistic code of their community. Prelinguistic communicative acts serve functions similar to those later expressed linguistically, indicating a continuity from preverbal to verbal communication. Knowledge of the development of interaction and communication patterns prior to the onset of speech is important in order to understand the acquisition of language. Some language-disordered children may not have developed communication skills that are prerequisites to learning language. The clinician needs to recognize what patterns of behavior precede language so that these prerequisite skills can be included in therapy programs for certain language-disordered children.

preintentional interactions

Although infants' early actions usually are reflexive, parents attribute meanings to many infant behaviors. In an effort to share experiences with their child, they behave as though the infant were an intentional partner in a social interchange. Parents often trigger reflexive actions and treat them as though they were the infant's purposeful responses. For example, a parent may touch the infant's cheek, causing reflexive mouth movements that resemble smiling. The parent often reacts as though the child were smiling as an intentional social act. Lewis (1978) states that these parent-initiated interactions introduce infants into an "interaction mode" of behavior and provide a context in which they learn that their actions have an effect on people and objects.

Attention to a common referent is a goal of parent-infant interactions from early in life and is a necessary prerequisite to communication and language learning. Parents' early attempts to gain the infant's attention include vocal and nonvocal behaviors to which infants are most responsive. Parents typically vocalize to infants in a higher pitched voice, with exaggerated intonation patterns, and with altered speed and rhythm (Sachs 1978; Stern 1977) These characteristics of vocalization, seemingly intuitively employed by parents, correspond with infants' early perceptual sensitivities (Sachs 1978). Nonvocal behaviors used to capture the child's attention include exaggerated facial expressions, head movements, gaze, and positioning the child face to face with the parent (Stern 1977). Vocalizations often accompany nonvocal attention-getting actions, providing opportunities for children to integrate vocal and nonvocal input in a social context.

Until three to four months of age, infants' attention seldom extends beyond themselves (Ginsburg and Opper 1979). Adapting to the capabilities of the child, parents limit the subject of their input to the infant's body and actions. They comment on or imitate the infant's hand movements; they touch the infant's feet and make some noise during kicking activities; they imitate or otherwise respond to mouth movements or vocalizations. Parents attend to the child's interests and behaviors in an effort to establish mutual activities.

When infants are about three months old, infant-parent coaction patterns begin (Stern and others 1978). Mutual gaze, posture sharing, and covocalizations are common during the three to four month age period. These joint activities serve an emotional bonding function and encourage the infant to share experiences with another person. Coactions frequently are structured into play routines which hold the child's attention and incorporate behaviors later used in more advanced communicative activities (Sachs 1978; Stern 1977; Bruner 1978). Facial expressions, eye contact, head movements, and vocalizing are used to initiate, interrupt, and terminate joint behaviors. Both the infant and the caregiver can exercise control over these interactions, and either may be required to adjust their actions to accommodate fluctuations in the other's behavior (Stern 1977; Bruner 1978). Turn taking, adjusting behavior to meet the needs of another, and use of behaviors to initiate, maintain, and terminate interactions are early routines into which dialogic exchanges later are incorporated. These joint activities are primitive forms of the interactional communicative function (Stern and others 1978) (see p. 22).

Initially, infants participate in covocalizing only if the parent vocalizes first and the infant joins the activity (Morehead and Morehead 1974; Stern and others 1978). This makes parents primarily responsible for initiating the shared activity. However, that infants influence the maintenance of these interactions is illustrated by the fact that parents cease vocalizing if the infant remains silent (Stern and others 1978). This represents an early instance of mutual feedback during vocal activities, an important prerequisite to language learning.

Between four and eight months of age, infants increasingly perceive their actions in relationship to the effects on the external environment (Morehead and Morehead 1974; Ginsburg and Opper 1979). They begin to repeat actions in an effort to recreate results, and they learn to differentiate between themselves and others and between an object and its movement or location. These are the perceptual prerequisites for subsequent differentiation between actors and actions, initiators and recipients of actions, and objects or events and their locations. They are the precursors to later development of semantic concepts expressed as agents, actions, patients, and locations, and of interactional skills necessary for successful use of language in social interchanges.

As infants recognize that other people's actions are separate from their own and that their actions affect other people and objects, caregivers and infants more frequently engage in alternate exchanges. Initially the parent must imitate the infant's acts in order to get the infant to repeat them. Subsequently, the infant will imitate the parent's behavior without having produced it immediately before the parent did, provided that the pattern is one the infant has produced before, that is, the behavior is in his or her repertoire (Morehead and Morehead 1974). As with coactions, parents at first assume the primary responsibility for maintaining alternate interchanges, often taking their role and that of the infant if the infant fails to respond in turn (Snow 1977). Parents provide input, pause for the infant's response, then act in the infant's place if he or she does not respond. Stern (1977) describes such events as "a monologue by the mother in the form of an imaginary dialogue" (p. 16). As infants begin to take their turn, a parent less often assumes their role, gradually shifting to them more responsibility for maintaining the interaction. These alternate response sequences have characteristics seen later in more advanced communicative acts.

Stern and others (1978) discuss the relationship between social context and the use of coactions and alternate actions early in the child's life. Covocalizations predominate during the infant's high-arousal states and generally are associated with emotions. Alternate patterns occur more frequently in midlevels of arousal and are used by parents in an instructional sense. Similar patterns continue in adulthood, when covocalizing is used most often in situations of extreme affect, while alternate exchanges characteristically are employed when information is exchanged. This suggests a continuity from infancy to adulthood in relationships between vocalization patterns and the situation as well as in the relationships between partners in vocal interactions.

In concert with infants' increased attention to objects and events separate from themselves, parents increase their efforts to direct attention to objects and activities external to the infants (Snow 1977). They mark or indicate the focus of attention by moving objects, placing objects near the child in a tempting manner, creating sound near the item of focus, and directional gesturing. Soon after four months of age, infants show recognition of another person's line of regard and begin visual cross-checking to determine whether they are focusing on the item of someone else's attention (Bruner 1978). Learning to follow another's line of attention serves as the initial basis for you/I distinctions and for use of linguistic structures to indicate place in later dialogue (Bruner 1978).

Parents report that after the infant is four to six months of age, they can differentiate cries for attention from vocalizations indicating pleasure or satisfaction (Bruner 1978). They state that the nature of their responses to the child's vocalizations is based on their interpretation of his or her intent. As a result of parents' responsiveness, infants begin to expect a response. Once a response expectancy pattern is established, infants show an insistence in calling, a reduction in the length of the call followed by a pause while awaiting a response, and a progressive stylization in the nature of the call. Such behaviors suggest that the infant is learning to initiate vocalizations to accomplish something. Bruner refers to this as acquiring the "demand mode" of communication.

Until about six months of age, infants vocalize as a part of total action schemes. Vocalizations seldom occur as isolated acts (Stern and others 1978). Action schemes, of which vocalizations are a part, reflect the infant's feelings and responses to external conditions but are not produced with the intent of representing such feelings (Bloom and Lahey 1978). Bates (1976) considers these preintentional actions to be perlocutionary acts, (see p. 19) since they bring about an interpretative response from another person. They are not illocutionary acts (see p. 19) because they are not produced with an intent to communicate.

During the sixth and seventh months of life, infants begin to produce a greater variety of sounds and to practice them repeatedly (Stern 1977).

Parents frequently imitate the infant's babbling, incorporating vocal behavior into social routines. While the infant does not engage in reduplicative babbling with the intent to communicate, the use of this vocal behavior in interactions with parents provides experience in including vocalizations in a social context. Bradley (1978) notes that infants often engage in reduplicative babbling when alone and proposes that this may be the initial appearance of self-reinforcement in the language learning process. It also is a forerunner of the imaginative function of language (see p. 23).

intentional interactions

Infants show a marked increase in intentional behaviors around eight to ten months of age. Before this time, they unintentionally cause something to happen and then repeat their actions in an effort to recreate results. They seem to recognize no cause of action other than their own (Piaget and Inhelder 1969). At about eight months, they begin to set their goal in advance and either select from old action schemes or attempt to discover new ones to achieve goals (Piaget and Inhelder 1969; Ginsburg and Opper 1969). This marks the beginning of the means-end distinction, which is necessary for subsequent learning of semantic relations and pragmatic functions.

During the eight to twelve month age period when infants recognize that other persons have actions separate from their own, they begin to use the "exchange mode" of interaction (Bruner 1978). The infant demands an object from someone (utilizing the previously learned "demand mode"), gives it back to the person, then demands it again. In this action sequence, infants experience role reversal, first serving as the recipient of an action, then as initiator, and again as the recipient. This serves as the basis for later learning of reciprocity in which there are specific rules for interchanges, as is the case in conversational exchanges (Bruner 1978). It also provides an experiential basis for subsequent learning of the agent, action, and object roles (Bruner 1975) (see p. 64) and of the deictic system (Rees 1978) (see p. 46).

With the differentiation between their own and another's actions and the recognition of means-end relationships, infants begin to employ other persons to assist in accomplishing a goal. This behavior generally emerges at ten to twelve months of age. Infants adopt novel means of communicating in an effort to reduce uncertainty in the outcome of their actions (Bruner 1978). Bell and Ainsworth (1972) point out that a parent's promptness in responding to infants' novel communicative behaviors encourages them to seek additional ways to communicate their intents. Where infants previously used crying as a principal mode for communicating, more specific acts, such as pointing and reaching, are employed to signal line of regard (Bruner 1978) and to convey intentions (Stark 1978). Bruner (1978) states that these behaviors reflect the establishment of "mutual recognition of a correct way to signal" (p. 32) and represent an initial step in conventionalization of communicative acts. He contends that the infant's learning to substitute new means to achieve more certain outcomes encourages subsequent learning of words to further reduce errors in interpretation of intent. Dore (1978) considers these actions as early forms of reference making in that they are used to indicate which items, events, or conditions are of immediate importance to the infant. Dore points out that these intentional referential behaviors have pragmatic functions but do not have propositional content. He therefore considers them to be communicative acts but not speech acts.

Bates (1976) calls the infant's early intentional behaviors illocutionary acts, since they are under the child's intentional control. She classifies as "protoimperatives" those acts performed intentionally by the infant to obtain a desired item. The infant's acts which are meant to direct the attention of others are classified as "protodeclaratives." Bates states that these are prototypes for linguistic imperatives and declaratives.

Children's expressions of intentions in the latter stages of prelinguistic development and in initial phases of language use are discussed further in this chapter in the section on the pragmatics of language. The continuity in development from preverbal to verbal behavior can be seen in that discussion on the functions of early communicative behaviors.

prelinguistic skills: examples of disordered development

Children with deficient communication abilities may fail to acquire skills that are prerequisites to language learning. Some give limited attention to their environment. They may not focus on objects or events going on around them. For example, novel sounds, movements, and human voices, all of which usually gain infants' attention, may go unnoticed. Children may continue to limit their attention to their own body movements and internal states long past the age at which this normally occurs. They may perform self-stimulating acts, such as rocking, producing gutteral sounds, or eye gouging, yet disregard external stimuli. Some children wander in a seemingly aimless fashion, not focusing on any particular object or activity for a sustained period of time. Without attention to their surroundings, children will not learn the interactional and communicative skills necessary for acquiring language.

Children with disorders in communication may show a reduced responsiveness to other people's efforts to interact with them. Infants may fail to respond to a parent's attempts to take part in activities which are of interest to the child. For example, infants' continuation or interruption of an activity, such as cooing, gazing, or moving their mouth or arms, may not be affected by whether their caregiver joins them in the activity. Another person's efforts to attract a child's attention may go unnoticed. For example, the child may not attend to parents' gazing, facial expressions, vocalizations, or posturing that is intended to draw the child's attention to them. The child may not follow other people's directional cues, such as gazing, pointing, or moving toward an external object or event. Children may fail to notice when the parent directs vocalizations, gestures, or speech to them as opposed to someone else. They may not learn conventional signals for directing someone else's attention, neither recognizing the intent when someone else performs directional acts nor learning to perform such acts to guide someone else's line of regard.

Children who are unaware that what they do affects people and objects with which they come in contact will not learn to use language for effective communication. Infants may fail to repeat an action in an effort to recreate results. For example, when infants kick their feet and the parent immediately thereafter moves their legs in a pleasing manner, infants usually learn quickly that they can cause the parent to move their legs by kicking their feet. They will repeat the action in an effort to bring about this result. A failure to repeat actions in an effort to cause something to recur suggests that children are not learning that what they do can bring about results. Infants or young children may fail to recognize that their demands bring about actions from other people and therefore not attempt to control what someone else does. They may not show a normal response expectancy by persisting in calling behaviors or by acting and then pausing to await the response. They may not try to prolong interactional episodes through actions that they have learned will cause another person to continue the interaction.

Some communicatively handicapped children show a preference for activities which do not include other people. They may choose to engage in activities alone rather than to participate with someone else. They may rarely attempt to entice someone to join them and even protest when another person intervenes. They may observe what others do but not interject themselves into the situation. Some children use other people as instruments to achieve a goal but do not include them as social partners.

Failure to learn routines associated with social interactions may indicate inadequate development of communication skills. Children may not show an anticipation of going somewhere when mother picks up the car keys. They may not learn alternate action routines, either in elementary turn-taking activities, such as alternate vocalizations, or in reciprocal activities, in which the actions of one person complement those of another. For example, they may not play games in which they drop something on the floor, someone else picks it up, and this sequence is repeated.

Some children do not adapt their behavior according to the context. Infants may not begin showing a preference for familiar over unfamiliar people at a normal age. They may not evidence appropriate reticence to perform socially for strangers or proceed with appropriate caution in unfamiliar activities.

Children with disordered language may not learn conventional ways to signal intent or meaning. They may continue to use very general signals, such as yelling, to indicate a variety of intents, failing to learn to alter what they do to reduce uncertainty in interpretation of their acts. They may not learn to interpret signals other people give for the purpose of influencing their behavior. For example, they may not recognize facial expressions or hand movements used by parents to signal approval or disapproval or to direct children's actions. Likewise, children may not learn to point or move toward an object to indicate line of regard or to look to the person whom they want to control. They may not learn that a parent whispers to signal that they should respond quietly. They may not use intonation, tone of voice, facial expressions, or posturing to indicate anger, happiness, rejection, or withdrawal.

Remediation programs for certain language-disordered children should focus on the prelinguistic abilities that are the forerunners to language learning. In working with infants and young children with deviant communication abilities, clinicians need to ensure that the prelinguistic skills that undergird language learning have been acquired before turning major efforts to teaching spoken language.

○ PRAGMATICS

People use language in social interchanges with other people. "Pragmatics refers to the study of the use of language in context, by real speakers and hearers in real situations" (Bates 1974, p. 277). The scope of information in a comprehensive study of the pragmatics of language is extensive and will not be covered in this book. For the present purpose of addressing language learning and language remediation for preschool children, attention will be focused on the communicative intents expressed through language and on certain aspects of the use of language in conversation.

expressing communicative intentions

Language serves both communicative and noncommunicative functions. Language produced with the intent of having an effect on another person serves a communicative function. Rees (1973) discusses the noncommunicative functions of language, which include the role of language in concept formation, in establishing self-image, in directing behavior, and in imaginative pursuits. While both the communicative and the noncommunicative functions will be considered in our discussion of normal and

Chap. 2 The Foundations for Language Intervention Programs 19

disordered language, greater attention will be focused on the communicative functions

People [perform] certain communicative acts when they speak to someone else. [They intend] for what they say to have particular effects on listeners. [Searle desc]ribes utterances used for communicating as "speech [acts":]

[Speaking a la]nguage is performing speech acts, acts such as making [statements,] commands, asking questions, making promises, and so [on; and more ex]actly, acts such as referring and predicating. (1969, p. [16])

[Searle lists four comp]onents of speech acts. *Utterance acts* are the [acts of uttering and ar]e a part of all speech acts. *Propositional acts* [involve referring and predicati]ng; they pertain to the conceptual content of [utterances. Illocutionary acts a]re the speakers' intended effects in speaking ([asserting, questioning, pr]omising, and so on). *Perlocutionary acts* are the [effects that the illocutio]nary acts have on the hearer (convincing, alarming, inspiring, and so on). Searle states that all speech acts include an utterance act (utter something), a propositional act (refer or predicate), and an illocutionary act (assert, direct, deny, and so on). A speech act may or may not have the intended perlocutionary force. In other words, it may or may not bring about the intended response from the listener.

It is important to differentiate a propositional from an illocutionary act. Dore (1975) explains:

> The proposition is essentially the conceptual content ... of the utterance, while the illocutionary force indicates how the utterance is to be taken or what the speaker's attitude is toward the proposition. (p. 30)

Searle (1969) states, "A proposition is what is asserted in the act of asserting, what is stated in the act of stating" (p. 29). Examples may help to clarify. In the statement *I admit that I lost your book,* the proposition is *I lost your book,* while the illocutionary act—admitting—is signaled by *I admit.* In the sentence *Shut the window!* the proposition is *Someone* (presumably an individual to whom the utterance is addressed) *shut the window.* The illocutionary force —commanding—is marked by intonation and sentence form and is interpretable within the context of the utterance. I will include the propositional component of speech acts in the discussion of the semantics of language.

Illocutionary acts are of primary importance in the consideration of language use. In producing an utterance, a speaker performs a certain act (warns, thanks, requests, indicates, and so on). The speaker's intended effect is the illocutionary force of the utterance. The act that is performed by uttering the sentence may be expressed explicitly (as in *I promise to send you the money"*) or implied (*I'll send you the money*). The speaker's intended effect often is not marked by the syntactic structure and is not revealed by a literal interpretation of the sentence. The intent generally can be interpreted only in light of the context of the utterance. The examples given in Table 2-1 illustrate that syntactic form and literal interpretation often do not express the illocutionary force of an utterance.

The term *performative* can be used to describe certain speech acts. Words which by their utterance accomplish the act they express or which are an actual part of the intended act are referred to as *explicit performatives* (Austin 1962) or *pure performatives* (Greenfield and Smith 1976). For example, one performs the act of promising by uttering the sentence *I promise to be there.* In that sentence, *promise* is an explicit performative. Greenfield and Smith (1976) contend that children use verbs such as *bye-bye* as pure performatives. They state, "Saying bye-bye to bid farewell is performing an act" (Greenfield and Smith 1976, p. 51). The word *bye-bye* in such a context has no propositional content; it has meaning as a part of the act being performed.

Analyzing utterances according to the speaker's objective in making the utterance (as illocutionary acts or performatives) represents a significant

TABLE 2-1
Examples of Illocutionary Acts

SITUATION	UTTERANCE	ILLOCUTIONARY ACT
In class, a girl searches in her purse (to no avail) for a pencil. Turning to a classmate, she says—	Do you have an extra pencil?	Requesting
When a woman answers a knock at the door, her neighbor says—	I'm out of salt.	Requesting
The plumbing in a man's apartment has broken. His guest says—	Why don't you call the owner?	Recommending
After watching the late news, a person says to her companion—	Aren't you sleepy?	Suggesting
When speaking to a large group in a warm room, the speaker says—	Will those windows open?	Requesting or recommending
When a prospective renter is being shown office space, she says to the real estate representative—	Will those windows open?	Inquiring
Upon receiving flowers from a friend, a woman says—	You were kind to bring these.	Thanking
In speaking to her young child, a mother says—	Put your toys in the toy box.	Commanding
After knocking his brother off the bicycle, the boy says—	I didn't mean to hurt you.	Apologizing
When mother enters the room where a vase is broken, the little girl says—	I didn't break it.	Denying

departure from traditional analyses of syntactic structure and propositional content of utterances. It focuses attention on the purposes for which language is used in context rather than on the linguistic structure or the conceptual content expressed within an utterance.

Expressing Intentions: Normal Development The functional nature of children's early nonverbal and verbal communicative acts received increasing attention in the study of child language during the 1970s. Pylyshyn (1977) states that the impetus to learn language comes from the child's intention to signal some meaning. Halliday (1977) purports that for a child, learning language is "the learning of a system of meanings" and that meanings refer "to the functions that language is made to serve in the life of a growing child" (p. 8).

Bates, Camaioni, and Volterra (1975), Bruner (1975, 1978), and Bates (1976) contend that the child's prelinguistic acts performed to communicate some intention are precursors to the expression of intent through language. Bates (1976) reports that at about ten to twelve months of age, a child learns certain performative functions which are expressed through vocal and gestural acts whose meanings are interpretable within the context of their utterance. For example, turning away from mother as she approaches with a cup may be a child's way of signaling rejection. Bates states:

> ... these early performatives might best be described as action schemes, procedural blueprints containing the communicative goal, the identity of the intended listener, and the kinds of signals that can be used to reach both. (Bates 1976, p. 433).

Children's early communicative acts can be described as having illocutionary force, since they are produced for the purpose of having particular effects on another person. Prelinguistic communicative acts have neither identifiable propositional content nor linguistic form, but they are performed with certain intents that later are encoded linguistically.

Greenfield and Smith (1976) suggest that children's early words are performatives rather than symbols with referential or propositional meanings. They note that pure performatives are common in children's early utterances. The example cited earlier of the young child's use of *bye-bye* while waving as a part of the act of bidding farewell illustrates the use of a pure performative. Similarly, saying "no" while turning away from something may be a part of the act of rejecting.

Bloom (1970) and Brown (1973) emphasize the necessity of considering the child's utterance in light of its context in order to interpret the child's intent. A word or sentence may perform different functions in different situations. For example, children may say "puppy" either to direct the parent's attention to the presence of a dog or to command someone to give them the puppy. When children begin talking, a listener must rely on their gestures, intonation, and relevant situational clues to recognize the intended meaning. However, when interpreted within their context, children's utterances express a variety of intents, even at the single-word level of production. In other words, children use language from the beginning to accomplish different purposes.

Classification systems for describing young children's communicative acts according to their function or to the illocutionary force of an utterance provide a framework for considering the development of communicative intent. Such systems also can be of assistance in planning assessment and remediation programs for children who use communicative acts for a restricted range of purposes. Halliday (1977) provides a classification system for the functional components of child and adult language. Dore, Gearhart, and Newman (1978) suggest a system for describing the illocutionary force of a young child's speech acts. The classifications used by Halliday and by Dore, Gearhart, and Newman will be discussed as examples of ways in which children's utterances can be considered according to their communicative function or purpose.

Halliday (1977) describes a functional basis for language and suggests that the components of early communication are transformed into the adult system of language. Based on his own child's patterns of development, he proposes three phases of development and identifies the components that emerge in each. Halliday explains that the functions learned early are generalized into more abstract functions in later phases. Table 2–2 summarizes Halliday's three-phase classification system.

In Phase I, occupying the period from about ten to eighteen months of age for Halliday's child, children learn a system of vocal and gestural acts which are meaningful in the situation in which they are used. These acts may not have linguistic form or propositional content, but they are meaningful in that they are effective in influencing the behaviors of others in ways that children intend. During Phase I, children's communicative acts serve the following functions:

> *Instrumental function:* Children use communicative acts as a means of satisfying their material needs and desires. When performing an instrumental act, who satisfies their needs is not important. The intended effect is to obtain the desired goods or services.
>
> *Regulatory function:* Children behave in certain ways for the purpose of controlling what someone else does. The regulatory function differs from the instrumental in that the intent is to control a particular individual rather than to obtain a particular item or service.
>
> *Interactional function:* Communicative behaviors performed for the purpose of interacting with another person are said to serve an interactional function. Acts fulfilling this role include greetings, efforts to establish joint attention, and attempts to draw another person into joint activities.

TABLE 2-2

Functional Components of Communication

Phase I	
Instrumental Function	Acts intended to satisfy material needs; the "I want" function
Regulatory Function	Acts intended to control other people; the "Do as I tell you" function
Interactional Function	Acts intended to establish interactions with other people; the "Me-you" function
Personal Function	Acts intended to express self; the "Here I come" function
Heuristic Function	Acts used to explore and organize the environment; the "Tell me why" function
Imaginative Function	Acts which create an imaginary environment; the "Let's pretend" function
Phase II	
Pragmatic Function	Language used to act on the environment
Mathetic Function	Language used to learn about the environment
Information Function	Language used to provide others with new information
Phase III	
Ideational Function	Language used to represent one's world
Interpersonal Function	Language used to participate in the world
Textual Function	Language used to express meanings through verbal symbols

Personal function: Communicative acts serve the personal function when their purpose is the expression of one's self. This function is evidenced in children's expressions of their feelings, attitudes, and interests.

Heuristic function: Children use language as a means of exploring and organizing their environment. This function may be noticed first when the child asks the name of things.

Imaginative function: When children use language to create an environment of their own, language is serving the imaginative function. This is seen initially when children create a world of "pure sound" and later in story telling and imaginative play.

For a given function, there are sets of alternative meanings. For example, Halliday's child, Nigel, expressed two meanings for the regulatory function. "Do that again" was one meaning, while "Do that right now," expressed with urgency, was a second. Nigel used a total of twelve meanings within the set of functions in Phase I, yet he expressed only one function by a single communicative act.

Children begin the transition from their own to adult language in Phase II, which for Nigel extended from about eighteen to twenty-four months of age. They begin using language not only to act on the environment but also to learn about it. The functions associated with Phase II are:

Pragmatic function: This function has its origin in the earlier learned instrumental and regulatory functions, with the interactional function also contributing to its acquisition. Children's use of words as actions is their use of language in a pragmatic sense. The child's learning of and differentiating between the pragmatic function and the mathetic function (described in the next paragraph) mark a transition toward the adult language system.

Mathetic function: Children's use of language for the purpose of learning about their environment is called the mathetic function. This grows out of the personal and heuristic functions, with the previously learned interactional function contributing. Language used to comment on, recall, or predict the existence of entities or the occurrence of events is mathetic. Halliday states that the mathetic function assists the child in learning about people, entities, and situations, and thus in constructing reality.

Informative function: Well after children have learned to employ language for the previously mentioned purposes, they learn that it can be used to provide other people with new information. Halliday stresses that children do not begin using language to inform until considerably after they use it for the previously mentioned functions. Halliday states that this is "the only purely intrinsic function of language, the only use of language in a function that is definable solely by reference to language" (1977, p. 21). He points out that while adults often consider this to be the major function of language, it is not the predominant function for young children.

During Phase II, children's communicative acts often have linguistic form. Many new words are learned to express previously learned functions. Nelson (1973) states that some children initially tend to use words primarily to name (mathetically), while others more often use words to interact (pragmatically). Halliday (1977) suggests that the pragmatic function encourages the development of syntax and the mathetic function promotes vocabulary growth.

Halliday (1977) states that a child's acquisition of words in Phase II permits a single utterance to serve more than one function, that is, to mean more than one thing. This is an important step toward mastery of the adult linguistic system, in which most utterances are multifunctional. During Phase II, children also begin to participate in dialogic exchanges when they are learning syntax. Dialogue requires the child to adopt and assign roles to participants in a conversation and to use linguistic forms in personal interactions. Learning to enter into dialogue is a necessary prerequisite for the acquisition of the informative and interpersonal functions.

The transition into Phase III marks children's entry into the adult linguistic system. For Halliday's child, this occurred at about twenty-four months of age. The major components of Phase III are:

Ideational function: This function, which arises from the mathetic function, is described as "... the observer function, language as a means of talking about the real world" (Halliday 1977, p. 17). This is the representational, cognitive function of language. It allows speakers to represent verbally their awareness of phenomena in the world.

Interpersonal function: The pragmatic function, learned in Phase II, is transformed into the interpersonal function, which is the use of language to take part in or to act on the world. Speakers use language in an interpersonal sense to project themselves into communicative situations and to attempt to have certain effects on listeners.

Textual function: This component creates the text of language. Of the textual function, Rees (1978) states, "It is meanings encoded into words or sentences" (p. 254). Halliday (1977) considers it to be "an enabling function" because its existence is necessary in order for the ideational and interpersonal components to be put to use.

Halliday states that the mathetic-pragmatic distinction in Phase II gives rise to the ideational-interpersonal distinction in Phase III. He reports that this separation of language to represent experiences (ideational) and language to interact socially (interpersonal) is at the base of the adult language system. The textual component is a necessary part of all utterances, since it creates the text.

Halliday (1977) emphasizes that ". . . the adult linguistic system is in fact founded on a functional plurality" (p. 52). Most utterances of adults have an ideational and an interpersonal component in that they express experiential meanings and are intended to have an effect on other people. While the uses of language by adults are many, most utterances have their basis in the ideational and interpersonal functions.

Dore, Gearhart, and Newman (1978) propose a system for defining children's utterances according to their illocutionary force. Their system was found to be a reliable means of coding the conversational acts (C-acts) of three year olds in conversations with peers and with the teacher in a nursery school setting. Of their system, Dore, Gearhart, and Newman state, "It is essentially an illocutionary model (as distinct from a grammatical or social one), in that a class of illocutionary acts are postulated as the primary units of conversation" (1978, p. 339).

Dore, Gearhart, and Newman identify three primary functions of children's utterances: to *convey content*, to *regulate the conversation*, and to *express attitudes*. For these three primary functions, they identify six general conversational classes. *Requestives, assertives, performatives,* and *responsives* are general classes that serve the primary function of conveying content. *Regulatives* fulfill the primary function of regulating conversation. *Expressives* serve the primary function of expressing attitudes. The general conversational classes are comprised of specific conversational acts (C-acts), which were used to classify the children's utterances. Table 2–3 identifies and defines the C-acts and provides examples of utterances classified under each. Figure 2–1 shows the relationships between the particular C-acts, their general conversational classes, and their primary conversational function.

TABLE 2–3

Codes, Definitions, and Examples of Conversational Acts

Code	Definition and Example
	Requestives solicit information or actions.
RQCH	*Choice Questions* seek either-or judgments relative to propositions: "Is this an apple?"; "Is it red or green?"; "Okay?"; "Right?"
RQPR	*Product Questions* seek information relative to most wh-interrogative pronouns: "Where's John?"; "What happened?"; "Who?"; "When?"
RQPC	*Process Questions* seek extended descriptions or explanations: "Why did he go?"; "How did it happen?"; "What about him?"
RQAC	*Action Requests* seek the performance of an action by hearer: "Give me it!"; "Put the toy down!"
RQPM	*Permission Requests* seek permission to perform an action: "May I go?"
RQSU	*Suggestions* recommend the performance of an action by hearer or speaker both: "Let's do it!"; "Why don't you do it?"; "You should do it."
	Assertives report facts, state rules, convey attitudes, etc.
ASID	*Identifications* label objects, events, people, etc.: "That's a car."; "I'm Robin."; "We have a boat."
ASDC	*Descriptions* predicate events, properties, locations, etc. of objects or people: "The car is red."; "It fell on the floor."; "We did it."
ASIR	*Internal Reports* express emotions, sensations, intents and other mental events: "I like it."; It hurts."; "I'll do it."; "I know."
ASEV	*Evaluations* express personal judgments or attitudes: "That's good."
ASAT	*Attributions* report beliefs about another's internal state: "He does not know the answer."; "He wants to."; "He can't do it."
ASRU	*Rules* state procedures, definitions, "social rules," etc.: "It goes in here."; "We don't fight in school."; "That happens later."
ASEX	*Explanations* state reasons, causes, justifications, and predictions: "I did it because it's fun."; "It won't stay up there."
	Performatives accomplish acts (and establish facts) by being said.
PFCL	*Claims* establish rights for speaker: "That's mine."; "I'm first."
PFJO	*Jokes* cause humorous effect by stating incongruous information, usually patently false: "We throwed the soup in the ceiling."
PFTE	*Teases* annoy, taunt, or playfully provoke a hearer: "You can't get me."
PFPR	*Protests* express objections to hearer's behavior: "Stop!"; "No!"
PFWA	*Warnings* alert hearer of impending harm: "Watch out!"; "Be careful!"

Chap. 2 The Foundations for Language Intervention Programs   27

As is shown in Table 2–3, *requestives* include C-acts which are choice, product, or process questions; action or permission requests; and suggestions for performing an action. *Assertives* include identifications and descrip-

TABLE 2–3 (continued)

Code	Definition and Example
	Responsives supply solicited information or acknowledge remarks.
RSCH	*Choice Answers* provide solicited judgments of propositions: "Yes."
RSPR	*Product Answers* provide Wh-information: "John's here."; "It fell."
RSPC	*Process Answers* provide solicited explanations, etc.: "I wanted to."
RSCO	*Compliances* express acceptance, denial, or acknowledgement of requests: "Okay."; "Yes."; "I'll do it."
RSCL	*Clarification Responses* provide solicited confirmations: "I said no."
RSQL	*Qualifications* provide unsolicited information to requestive: "But I didn't do it."; "This is not an apple."
RSAG	*Agreements* agree or disagree with prior non-requestive act: "No, it is not."; "I don't think you're right."
RSAK	*Acknowledgments* recognize prior non-requestives: "Oh."; "Yeah."
	Regulatives control personal contact and conversational flow.
ODAG	*Attention-Getters* solicit attention: "Hey!"; "John!"; "Look!"
ODSS	*Speaker Selections* label speaker of next turn: "John"; "You."
ODRQ	*Rhetorical Questions* seek acknowledgment to continue: "Know what?"
ODCQ	*Clarification Questions* seek clarification of prior remark: "What?"
ODBM	*Boundary Markers* indicate openings, closings and shifts in the conversation: "Hi!"; "Bye!"; "Okay"; "Alright"; "By the way"
ODPM	*Politeness Markers* indicate ostensible politeness: "Please"; "Thank you"
	Expressives non-propositionally convey attitudes or repeat others.
EXCL	*Exclamations* express surprise, delight or other attitudes: "Oh!"; "Wow"
EXAC	*Accompaniments* maintain contact by supplying information redundant with respect to some contextual feature: "Here you are"; "There you go"
EXRP	*Repetitions* repeat prior utterances.
	Miscellaneous Codes
UNTP	*Uninterpretables* for uncodable utterances.
NOAN	*No Answers* to questions, after 2 seconds of silence by addressee.
NVRS	*Non-verbal Responses* for silent compliances and other gestures.

From Dore, J., M. Gearhart, and D. Newman, The structure of nursery school conversation. In K. Nelson (ed.), *Children's Language, Vol. 1*. New York: Gardner Press, 1978, pp. 371–372. Reprinted by permission.

```
Primary                General              Particular
Conversational         Conversational       Conversational
Function               Class                Act
```

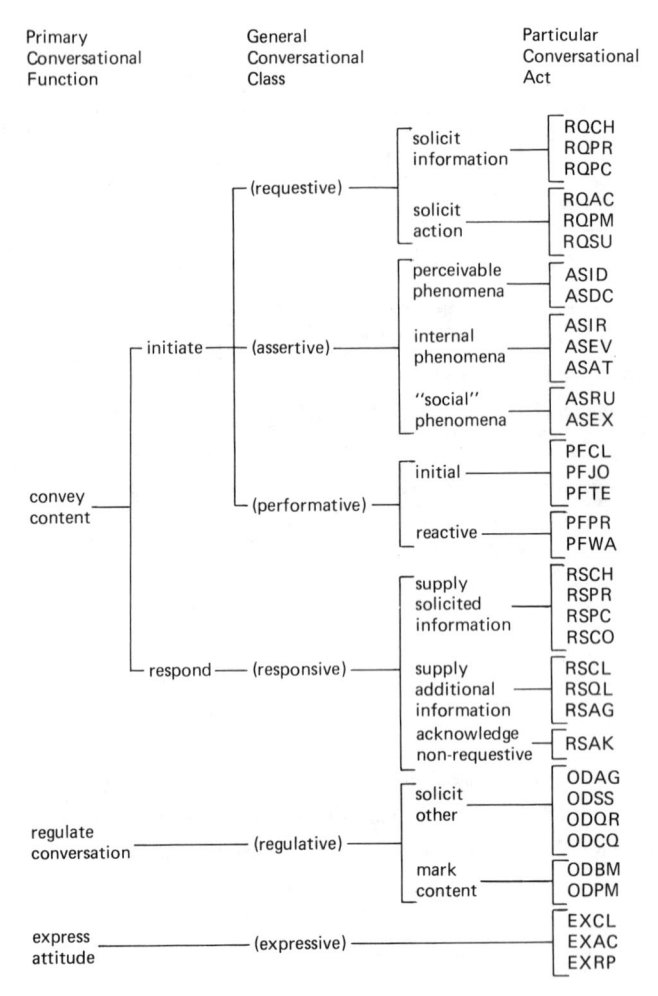

```
                                      ┌─ solicit          ┌─ RQCH
                                      │  information      ├─ RQPR
                                      │                   └─ RQPC
                      ┌─ (requestive) ┤
                      │               │                   ┌─ RQAC
                      │               │  solicit          ├─ RQPM
                      │               └─ action           └─ RQSU
                      │
                      │                   ┌─ perceivable  ┌─ ASID
                      │                   │  phenomena   └─ ASDC
                      │                   │
                      │                   │               ┌─ ASIR
          ┌─ initiate ┼─ (assertive) ─────┤  internal     ├─ ASEV
          │           │                   │  phenomena    └─ ASAT
          │           │                   │
          │           │                   │  "social"     ┌─ ASRU
          │           │                   └─ phenomena    └─ ASEX
          │           │
          │           │                                   ┌─ PFCL
convey    │           │                   ┌─ initial ─────┤ PFJO
content ──┤           └─ (performative) ──┤               └─ PFTE
          │                               │
          │                               │  reactive     ┌─ PFPR
          │                               └─              └─ PFWA
          │
          │                               ┌─ supply       ┌─ RSCH
          │                               │  solicited    ├─ RSPR
          │                               │  information  ├─ RSPC
          │                               │               └─ RSCO
          │                               │
          └─ respond ── (responsive) ─────┤  supply       ┌─ RSCL
                                          │  additional ──┤ RSQL
                                          │  information  └─ RSAG
                                          │
                                          │  acknowledge
                                          └─ non-requestive ─ RSAK

                                          ┌─ solicit       ┌─ ODAG
                                          │  other         ├─ ODSS
regulate                                  │                ├─ ODQR
conversation ────────── (regulative) ─────┤                └─ ODCQ
                                          │
                                          │  mark          ┌─ ODBM
                                          └─ content       └─ ODPM

express                                                    ┌─ EXCL
attitude ────────────── (expressive) ──────────────────────┤ EXAC
                                                           └─ EXRP
```

FIGURE 2–1 A network representation of the primary conversational functions, general classes, and particular conversational acts in the coding scheme.
From Dore, J., M. Gearhart, and D. Newman. The structure of nursery school conversation. In K. Nelson (ed.), *Children's Language, Vol. I.* New York: Gardner Press, 1978, p. 374. Reprinted by permission.

tions of objects, events, people, locations, and so on; reports of one's own internal states and the perceived internal conditions of others; evaluative statements; statements of rules governing procedures, social interactions, and so on; and explanations of reason, cause, justification, and prediction. Utterances which report facts, give rules, convey attitudes, and explain the reasons for conditions or acts are classified as assertives. *Performatives* are utterances which accomplish deeds or establish facts by their very utterance. Claims, jokes, teases, protests, and warnings all are considered to be performatives. *Responsives* are utterances which give answers, explanations, or judgments specifically sought by preceding questions or statements; provide additional but unsolicited information; and acknowledge prior utterances which do not request a response. *Regulatives* are utterances which control the flow of conversation and maintain social contact with a conversational partner. Often they do not have significant propositional content. Regulatives include utterances which gain the attention of the intended hearer; identify the person who is to speak next; mark conversational turns; seek clarification of a previous utterance; and convey politeness. *Expressives* are nonpropositional utterances which express attitudes, such as surprise, excitement, or dislike; maintain contact with another person by giving information that is redundant with some contextual information or condition; or repeat prior utterances.

Dore, Gearhart, and Newman found that some utterances required double coding, since it was not possible to determine unequivocally the child's intent in making the utterance. However, through the use of decisions procedures which were applied to all utterances, most utterances could be classified as a particular C-act.

The studies by Halliday (1977) and Dore, Gearhart, and Newman (1978) show that children's early communicative acts serve a variety of functions or express an identifiable set of intents. They provide examples of categories which can be used for describing children's communicative behaviors from these perspectives. Different categories have been used in other studies of pragmatic intentions expressed by young children (Dore 1975, 1977; Curtiss, Prutting, and Lowell 1979). The categories for describing the communicative functions and intents of children's utterances are sure to be revised with additional research and expansions in application of such classification systems. However, persons concerned with language disorders of young children can use the Halliday and the Dore, Gearhart, and Newman systems, or some revision thereof, as a framework for looking at functional communication skills and for establishing goals and procedures for assisting children in learning to use language effectively.

Expressing Intentions: Examples of Disordered Development

Children with language disorders may be restricted communicatively because they use language for a limited variety of purposes. They may perform communicative acts to get something they want but not to regulate other people, learn about their environment, or express their feelings and attitudes. They may not use language to explore and organize their environment, to test their hypotheses about the world, or to gain insights into the knowledge and beliefs of other people. Some children may use language only when they want additional information about a novel item or experience, or in describing events they engage in or observe. They may not recognize that language can assist them in interacting with other people, in influencing someone else's actions, or in becoming a part of others' activities Children may not progress normally in language learning because they do not know how to use language to accomplish important purposes.

To date, formal studies of communicative intents expressed by language-disordered children are few. Snyder (1975, 1978) found that young children with language disorders, when compared with a group of normal children matched by mean length of utterance (MLU), were deficient in the use of declarative and imperative performatives. Rees (1978) reports that Geller and Wollner (1976) found that language-disordered children between three and five years of age expressed a limited number of communicative intents. Curtiss, Prutting, and Lowell (1979) reported that preschool children with impaired hearing expressed a variety of pragmatic intentions nonverbally, but they frequently lacked the linguistic abilities necessary for encoding these intentions. Blank, Gessner, and Esposito (1979) present a case study of a three year old whose language was near normal in content and form but extremely delayed in terms of language use. Not only was he unable to use language as an effective communication device, he also had very limited preverbal communicative skills. Rom and Bliss (1981) found that compared to normal-speaking age peers, language-disordered children, like normal speakers matched for MLU, used significantly fewer utterances that served descriptive and acknowledging functions and more utterances that served an answering function. They did not differ from age peers or from speakers of comparable MLU in use of utterances serving interjecting, repeating, requesting-an-answer, practicing, self-expressing or protesting functions.

Examples from the author's clinical experiences illustrate restrictions in the scope of purposes which language serves for some language-disordered children.

> Margie, age four, produced many intelligible utterances which she used primarily for obtaining items or services. She gestured toward toys and food she wanted, often saying the name of the item as she pointed. Her mother reported that at home, Margie would hit the refrigerator door and say "juice," gesture or look toward a toy out of her reach and say the name of the toy, or look out the back door toward her swing set and say "swing" when she wanted someone to open the door so that she could go outside to play. Most of Margie's words referred to items she used or wanted or to activities in which she liked to engage, and she uttered these words as requests or demands for items or assistance. Margie did not refer to people by name. She was selective about who fulfilled her desires only at night when someone rocked her before she went to bed or when unfamiliar people tried to interact directly with her. Margie indicated a preference for her mother's rocking her at bedtime by leading her mother to the rocking chair. If she was unable to find her mother when she was among strangers, she cried. Margie did not verbalize to indicate her preference for one person over another, to seek information, to comment on what she or someone else was doing, to engage other people in social interactions, or

to express her feelings. Her mother described her as "a quiet child." She reported that Margie played alongside other children, showed a sustained interest in watching her siblings play, and was easily enticed into nonverbal play routines with family members. However, she did not initiate social interactions.

Using Halliday's terminology, Margie's language usually served an instrumental function, and she performed a few nonlinguistic communicative acts which fulfilled regulatory and interactional functions. Margie used language to get things she wanted but rarely to establish social relationships or to learn about and organize her environment.

> Four-year-old Ron was a very social child who used linguistic and nonlinguistic communicative acts for interacting with other people. Typical of his utterances were "Look!" "Watch me," "Come here," "My turn," "Sit down," "Let's go," and "Wait." He used a variety of greetings, including "Hi," "Glad-to-see-you," and "Hey there," and he bid farewell with "Goodbye" and "So long." He referred to many people by name, and he was quick to pick up on verbal and nonverbal social routines. His parents reported, "He is a part of everything." He laughed when others laughed, even when he obviously did not understand the cause of the laughter. He furrowed his brow or scowled when others talked in angry tones or cried. He used exaggerated facial expressions to indicate surprise when an unexpected or sudden noise or activity occurred. His mother described him as "the neighborhood social director," explaining that he initiated interactions with everyone and often directed what others were to do. Ron's vocabulary was extremely limited. He knew the names of few items or actions. He did not use language, either when alone or in the presence of others, for commenting on or describing what he or someone else was doing, or for forecasting future events. Ron often asked for a person's name but not for the names of objects. When he wanted a certain item, he went to great lengths to get it for himself, but he never asked for it verbally.

For Ron, verbal and nonverbal communicative acts served certain pragmatic but rarely mathetic or informative functions. He used language for social interactions but not to get items he wanted or to structure and explore his surroundings. Using the categories proposed by Dore, Gearhart, and Newman, Ron's utterances would be classified primarily as regulatives and expressives, with a few considered as requestives and performatives.

> Paul, age five, rarely initiated or attempted to prolong interactions with other people either through verbal or nonverbal acts. Most of his unsolicited utterances, if directed to another person, were requests for information or for verification of his observations or predictions. When playing alone or observing what someone else was doing, Paul used complex utterances in giving detailed descriptions about his or someone else's actions or about objects in the environment. On the rare occasions when he attempted to ask for assistance, to regulate what someone else did, or to participate in social interchanges, his intents were difficult to interpret, and he frequently resorted to gestures or withdrew quickly from the interaction. In conversa-

tional exchanges, Paul's contributions often seemed unrelated to the other speaker's statements or questions unless he was asked for a specific bit of information, such as the label or function of an item or a description of an action. His parents reported that as a younger child, Paul began using words at a normal age but was somewhat late in producing multiword utterances. His parents and teacher expressed concern because he rarely played with other children. They reported that he appeared overwhelmed on occasions when he was supposed to be group leader and direct other children, when he needed to defend himself verbally, or when he was brought into situations involving imaginative play. They also reported that he rarely expressed emotions and that he seemed insensitive to the feelings of other people. His teacher described Paul as "intellectually capable," "analytical," "a loner," "not demanding," and "not imaginative or creative."

For Paul, language was primarily mathetic. He used language in an ideational but rarely in an interpersonal sense. By the Dore, Gearhart, and Newman categories, Paul's utterances would be classified primarily as requestives (usually choice, product, or process questions), assertives (usually identifications and descriptions), and responsives (usually choice, product, and process answers, with some qualifications, compliances, and acknowledgments). He rarely used utterances that would be classified as performatives, regulatives, or expressives. Paul used language to organize and explore his environment but infrequently to get what he wanted, to control other people, to establish or maintain social relationships, or to express his own feelings and attitudes.

Margie, Ron, and Paul each present deficits in language use. For them, language serves a restricted range of purposes, and they experience breakdowns in communication because of these deficits. Other children with disordered language will reveal different patterns of limitations in using language to serve various functions and to express different intentions. For children who have not learned to use language as a mechanism for accomplishing an appropriate range of purposes, remediation programs designed to expand the functions which language can serve should be implemented.

language in conversation

Because language frequently is the medium through which people interact, it is important to consider how it is used in conversation. Grice (1975) proposes certain "Cooperative Principles" that participants in conversation assume will be followed:

> The quantity of what is said should be sufficient to convey the desired information but should not be excessive.
>
> Speakers should say what they have cause to believe is true.
>
> The information expressed should be relevant to the message being conveyed.

Speakers should organize what is said so that the message will not be ambiguous or obscure.

Listeners expect speakers to follow these principles or to make violations obvious to the listener. When a speaker intentionally violates a conversational principle and makes the violation overt, listeners recognize that the speaker does not intend the literal meaning of the statement, and they attempt to determine how the speaker meant the utterance to be taken. Listeners often interpret statements as ironic or humorous if violations of a conversational principle are obviously intentional. If the speaker violates a principle without overtly indicating that this has been done, listeners may be misled. The listener's efforts to figure out the speaker's intended meaning when a literal interpretation does not suffice are referred to as "conversational implicatures" (Grice 1975).

To be successful in conversation, participants must be sensitive to each other's needs and abilities. They must employ certain strategies to maintain the flow of conversation. They must determine what information relative to the topic of conversation is shared by those who are taking part; express what is not known or recognized by both the speakers and listeners if such information is essential for appropriate interpretation of what is said; and signal which information is assumed to be shared and which is new. They must adjust the form of their utterances so that it is appropriate and effective in its context. Speakers and listeners must learn and use the linguistic devices which orient the content of utterances relative to the time, location, and participants in conversation.

Maintaining the Flow of Conversation Basic to all conversation is turntaking. Conversational partners agree that they will not talk simultaneously, and they employ interpretable signals to indicate when they will initiate and terminate their roles as speaker or listener. Behaviors such as eye contact, nonsubstantive utterances as "oh" or "hmmm," facial expressions, and gestures such as nodding are common indicators that the message is or is not being received and understood. Mature speakers and listeners use language to maintain a common focus and to provide clarity and cohesion in conversation. Topic-relevant responses, linguistically contingent responses, pronominalizations, and grammatical ellipsis are among the devices used to maintain the flow of conversation (Bloom and Lahey 1978). If speakers or listeners have doubts about the topic, sequential questions or comments are used to clarify or to insure a common focus and interpretation.

Maintaining the Flow of Conversation: Normal Development

Children begin learning certain conventions that underlie conversation quite early. As was mentioned in the earlier section on Precursors to the Acquisition of Language, Bateson (1975), Snow (1977), Stern (1977), Bruner (1978), and others describe patterns of infant-parent interactions which they consider to be prototypes for conversation. Through joint activities with their parents, peers, and other persons, infants learn certain routines that later are transformed into conversational rules.

During the single-word stage of development, children observe several basic rules of conversation. They take turns speaking, and they frequently use verbal and nonverbal acts to gain the listener's attention. Young children may say "Look," "Hey," or "Uh-oh," or they may point, hold an object toward the intended listener, reach toward an object, or touch the intended listener before addressing the person. At about two years of age, children begin to call the name of the person whom they are addressing and to await a response before continuing with what they plan to say. Bloom and Lahey (1978) state that this is an early indication that children are starting to monitor conversational interactions.

Between two and three years of age, children begin accepting greater responsibility for maintaining dialogue. Keenan (1974) notes that at twenty-nine months of age, her twins had certain types of organization in their dialogues. When one twin directed a comment, question, or command to the other, he expected a response, even if it were nothing more than acknowledgment from the listener that the comments had been heard. Keenan's twins did not require a response to songs, narratives, or sound play, although the one in the role of listener often acknowledged that these had been received, seemingly in an effort to maintain the flow of the interchange.

Bloom, Rocissano, and Hood (1976) report that between two and three years of age, subjects in their study showed an increased effort to maintain the topic across conversational turns. The children began producing responses which preserved the topic of the speaker's prior utterance. Their earliest responses indicating topic sharing were repetition of all or part of the prior utterance:

> *Adult:* Let's pick up the toys now.
> *Child:* Pick up toys.

or additions of information to what had just been said:

> *Adult:* Tommy dropped his crayons.
> *Child:* Made a mess.

Before age three, the children rarely maintained the shared topic for more than two utterances.

Around age three, children begin producing more responses which are contingent linguistically on the prior utterance in an effort to achieve continuity in dialogue. Bloom, Rocissano, and Hood (1976) report that the three year olds in their study gave responses containing the same verb relations as the adult's prior utterance:

>   *Adult:* Bill broke something.
>   *Child:* Broke the cup.

Rodgon (1979) found that children whose mean utterance length ranged from 1.4 to 2.2 recognized yes/no and naming questions as verbalizations requiring a specific type of response. While the children did not always respond correctly to yes/no questions, they never gave a yes or no response to a naming question. One of Rodgon's subjects responded to questions which she did not appear to understand with utterances such as "hmmm?" or "huh?" Rodgon notes that such responses were "adaptive from the perspective of maintaining communicative give-and-take" (Rodgon 1979, p. 87).

At about three years of age, children begin using pronouns to provide cohesion in discourse (Bloom and Lahey 1978). Their response contains a pronoun referring back to a noun in the prior statement of the other speaker:

>   *Adult:* Did you eat your sandwich?
>   *Child:* I didn't want it.

or

>   *Adult:* Where is Jack?
>   *Child:* He's outside.

Pronouns used in this manner tie the response to the stimulus utterance, indicating that the second speaker's utterance is related to the first speaker's.

To achieve continuity across conversational turns, adults use grammatical ellipsis, whereby certain sentence constituents that are redundant with a prior utterance are deleted:

>   *First Speaker:* I enjoyed that movie.
>   *Second Speaker:* I didn't.

The second speaker deletes *enjoy that movie,* which is redundant with the prior utterance. Children do not begin using grammatical ellipsis in this manner until after three years of age (Bloom, Miller, and Hood 1975).

Based on a study of spontaneous narratives of three, four, and five year olds, Umiker-Sebeok (1979) provides insights into the conversational patterns of children in these age groups. The three year olds generally completed their narratives in a single conversational turn, not requiring the listener to respond. Children in this age group seldom preceded their narratives with an introduction intended to gain the listener's attention (*You know what?* or some summons to the intended listener). The three year olds did not attempt to engage in extended verbal exchanges pertaining to their own or another child's narratives.

Umiker-Sebeok found that the four and five year olds had an average of about one and one-half speaking turns per narrative. Most of the children in the older groups introduced their narratives with comments to gain the listener's attention. At four and five years of age, the children engaged in conversation relative to the narratives much more frequently and extensively than did the younger children. Increasingly, the structure of their utterances indicated efforts to influence the listener's interpretation of what they said, and they showed an increased reliance on others' responses to direct their continued explanations.

In summary, prior to the onset of speech, children learn certain interaction patterns which are prototypes of conversation. In the stage of single-word use, they observe certain basic rules of conversation, and they use linguistic and nonlinguistic acts to gain the listener's attention before they speak. Not until around age three do children show substantial increases in efforts to maintain dialogue. Near their third birthday, they begin expecting the addressees to acknowledge their statements, and they acknowledge statements of others in an attempt to maintain the flow of conversation. They also begin giving responses which are topically and then linguistically contingent on prior utterances, thereby achieving cohesion in dialogue. After age three, children learn to use grammatical ellipsis to provide cohesion across conversational turns.

Maintaining the Flow of Conversation: Examples of Disordered Development

Some children do not acquire normal interactional and communicative skills at a prelinguistic level of development and therefore are not prepared to learn to use language in conversation. Children with language disorders may have begun talking and expressing certain meanings through language yet not be successful participants in dialogue because they have not learned effective modes of interaction to which language can be applied. The development of these prelinguistic skills as well as behaviors which suggest breakdowns in their acquisition were discussed earlier in this book.

Children may learn to use language to make reference and issue propositions but fail to learn procedures for engaging in conversation. Such children generally are more successful if a monologue suffices than if the situation demands dialogue. Certain types of communication breakdowns may indicate that a child has not learned basic rules for conversational exchanges.

When children persistently interrupt another speaker or disregard someone's interrupting when they are speaking, they may not recognize the basic principles dictating that participants take turns talking in conversational episodes. Children who are not learning the rules of conversation may not understand or employ signals indicating that one is or is not willing to relinquish the floor when interrupted. For example, normally one stops talking while persons who interrupt say what they have to say, thus acknowledging the rule of taking turns. People may talk slightly louder or more rapidly to indicate they are not willing to relinquish their role as speaker, thereby discouraging the person who interrupts from continuing. Children who do not abide by the rules of turn-taking, either by discontinuing what they say when interrupted or by signaling in some way that they will not give up their role as speaker, may not have learned a basic rule of conversation.

Some children do not recognize that one should have the conversational partner's attention before speaking. A failure to use or respond to attention-getting signals may indicate a lack of knowledge of this conversational device. For example, children may employ neither the nonlinguistic attention-getting signals (touching, turning the addressee toward them, positioning themselves in front of the person to whom they are speaking, waving) nor the linguistic signals (*Hey! Look! Listen,* or calling the person's name) to insure that they have the attention of the individual to whom they are speaking. Likewise, they may not demonstrate an awareness that someone else's use of such signals is meant to get their attention, so they do not acknowledge being addressed. The behavior of a four-year-old child with delayed language illustrates a problem of this nature:

> Mr. S. expressed concern because he could not tell if his daughter was talking to him, a pet, her toys, her mother, or herself. The child did not indicate whom she was addressing by looking at the person, moving toward them, saying something to gain their attention, or any other discernible means. Mr. S. reported that the child would say the same thing repeatedly as she continued in her activity, never indicating vocally, nonvocally, or linguistically whom she was addressing. If addressees failed to respond when she was talking to them, the child became angry and cried. He also reported that the child indicated that she recognized when she was being addressed only if the speaker called her name or touched her. The child did not appear to recognize the significance of waving, gesturing, or using verbal indicators such as *Look* or *Hey* when these were used in an effort to gain her attention.

Some children with language disorders are not successful in conversation because they do not preserve the topic from the speaker's prior utterance. Attempting to converse with children whose responses do not seem to be related topically to the prior utterance often is confusing and may discourage continuation of the exchange. The behavior of a five-year-old language-disordered child reveals such a deficit in communication:

> Mrs. K. reported that attempts to carry on a conversation with her son usually were short-lived because of the nature of the child's participation. The mother stated, "When you say something to him, what he says back often seems to be about a completely different subject." She explained that the child carried out instructions and usually answered direct questions correctly, provided that they required only a short answer that was specifically asked for in the question. However, if someone made a comment to the child or asked an open-ended question, his follow-up statement frequently did not preserve the topic of the other speaker's prior utterance in a manner that was recognizable to other persons. As an example, Mrs. K. reported that when she picked up the child from school the previous day, she said, "We are going to get you some new sandals today." The child responded, "Bill spilled his juice." After extensive probing from her, the child finally indicated that Bill had worn new sandals to school that day. Mrs. K. explained that if she asked enough questions, she usually was able to determine that her son's responses were somehow related to what had been said to him, but the nature of his initial response did not reveal the relationship. This mother had concluded that her son "doesn't seem to realize that people stop talking to him because what he says back confuses them."

Some children with language disorders may maintain the basic topic across conversational turns but fail to use responses which are linguistically contingent. While responses which fail to match the prior utterance in linguistic form are not as confusing as those which appear unrelated topically, linguistic mismatches between a response and the preceding utterance tend to disrupt the flow of conversation. The following case suggests a deficit in the use of linguistically contingent responses in conversational exchanges:

> In describing the communication difficulties of a five-year-old boy in her class, a teacher cited an instance which she said typified conversational exchanges with the child. She asked the child, who was playing in the sandbox, "Where is the sand bucket?" He replied, "Susan did." In an effort to interpret his response, she looked around the play yard and saw that Susan had taken the bucket to another part of the yard. Only then was she able to see how the boy's response was related to her question.

The teacher's temporary confusion in interpreting the child's response would have been avoided had he used the appropriate linguistic form to match the question.

Presuppositions When speakers and listeners converse, what they say, how they say it, and how they interpret what is said is influenced by their ability to relate the propositional content of the utterance to their own and to the other's prior information and experiences. It is the speaker's responsibility to encode new information and whatever old information the listener must have in order to interpret and respond to statements appropriately. Speakers select the content and form of their sentences at least partially on the basis of their presuppositions about the relevant knowledge that the listener already possesses and according to their judgments of what the listener needs to know in order to make an appropriate interpretation and response.

Presuppositions can be described as *old, given,* or *prior* information, while the information not already known to the listener is the "new" information in a sentence. Mature speakers and listeners depend on certain conventions for marking *given* in contrast to *new* information. Clark and Haviland (1977) refer to this as the "given-new" contract agreed upon by discourse participants. They state:

> The given-new distinction . . . is present in language to serve a specific function. To ensure reasonably efficient communication, the speaker and listener adhere to a convention regarding the use of this distinction in sentences. The speaker tries, to the best of his ability, to make the structure of his utterances congruent with his knowledge of the listener's mental world. He agrees to convey information he thinks the listener already knows as given information and to convey information he thinks the listener doesn't yet know as new information. The listener, for his part, agrees to interpret all utterances in the same light. The result is what we have called the given-new contract . . . (Clark and Haviland 1977, p. 4)

Speakers and listeners rely on several sources of shared information. Accepting a sentence as appropriate may require knowledge or belief that the conditions referred to in the sentence are true. For example, the statement "I regret that you missed the party" presupposes that there was a party and that you did not attend. If either of these presuppositions is incorrect, the sentence is an inappropriate statement. The basis for presuppositions may be contained in a preceding sentence. In the sentence pair "I had pneumonia last week. I haven't yet fully recovered," interpretation of the second sentence presupposes the information in the first. Speakers and listeners can use the immediate nonverbal context as the shared information to which propositions are related. For example, the statement "They are cute" would be interpreted meaningfully by a listener who, with the speaker, is watching small puppies play. In a different setting, speakers would need to encode additional information to insure that the listener relates their statement to the appropriate set of circumstances. If addressing a person who shared the experience, the speaker might say "Those puppies were cute." For someone who had not seen the puppies, the speaker would need to include more background or given information and might say "The puppies in my backyard are cute." Presuppositions may not be stated if they are thought to be a part of the speaker's and the listener's shared knowledge of the world. A father's warning, "That limb is too small!" shouted to his daughter as she climbs higher in a tree, presupposes a shared knowledge that the size of a tree limb is related to its capability of supporting one's weight and of the consequences of placing one's weight on a limb that will not provide support. Unless this is shared knowledge, the daughter's interpretation of her father's statement is not likely to match his intent in issuing the warning.

In selecting the content and form for sentences, speakers are influenced by their awareness of cultural expectations and of their social role relative to the listener's. Stated differently, speakers choose the structure and content of an utterance at least partially on the basis of their judgments of what is the most socially appropriate way to encode a message in a particular situation. Bates (1976) refers to considerations of social context as a part of "pragmatic presuppositions." Examples will illustrate the impact of social relationships and contexts on utterance forms. Consider the context in which each of the following statements would be appropriate:

1. How dainty you look in that outfit.
2. Shut the stupid window!
3. Ms. Russell, please let me help you with that package.
4. You are a sissy!

Our cultural background and awareness of the effect of social role on linguistic form and content allow us to presuppose certain information about the speaker, the listener, and the situation in which these four statements would be appropriate. The speaker and listener in sentence 1 probably are both female, although the speaker could be a male addressing a female who is younger than he or with whom he is (or wishes to be) familiar. The statement likely would be made in a private or semiprivate situation rather than as an announcement before a large group. For sentence 2, the speaker probably is talking to a peer or someone younger, and the addressee likely is not a stranger. Such a statement would be made in an informal environment. Were the speaker addressing an older person, an authority figure, or a stranger, the utterance probably would be stated as "Please shut the window" or "Would you mind shutting the window." The form and content of sentence 3 suggest that the speaker is addressing a social superior (possibly a social equal) and that they are only casually acquainted or have a formal relationship. The speaker, most likely an adult, seems to be talking to someone older or possibly to a distinguished peer. Sentence 4 would be chosen for addressing a peer or someone younger and would not be appropriate in a formal setting. Both the speaker and listener probably are adolescent or younger.

Speakers can convey their messages either directly or with varying degrees of indirectness. Social role and interpersonal relationship between speakers and listeners, the setting of the communication episode, cultural expectations, speakers' intentions, and the participants' facility in using the linguistic system influence speaking style. The use of indirect forms generally reflects the speaker's efforts to be polite. Speakers are more likely to use indirect forms in addressing a person whom they perceive to be in a role of authority or held in high regard, in talking with strangers or others with whom they have only a superficial relationship, or in situations in which a formal rather than a casual interaction is appropriate. Speakers' selections of direct or indirect patterns of address are based at least partially on their presuppositions about their role and status relative to the listener and the nature of interaction appropriate in the immediate social context.

The prior discussion indicates that presuppositions have a significant influence on the content and form of what people say. The speaker and listener must share common factual knowledge and beliefs relative to the proposition if a sentence is to be interpreted as intended. To be successful in discourse, participants must make assumptions about their conversational partner's prior knowledge, capabilities, and expectations. In addition, certain social conventions must be considered in selecting linguistic form and content.

Presuppositions: Normal Development

To be successful in conversational exchanges, children need to learn what to say as well as what not to say if they are to communicate effectively in various situations. They must learn to anticipate what information the listener has and needs in order to understand what is said. Children need to learn social rules which determine how one should phrase a proposition so that it will be socially appropriate in a particular context. Brown (1973) addresses the child's learning task in the following statement:

> A sentence well adapted to its function is, like a piece in a jigsaw puzzle, just the right size and shape to fit the opening left for it by local conditions and community understandings. The child has to learn to adapt the size and complexity of his sentences to changing situations and interlocutors. (p. 168)

Greenfield and Smith (1976) suggest that in the single-word stage of development, children demonstrate some recognition of the given information-new information distinction. They generally encode whatever is undergoing change or is unusual (new information) instead of constant conditions in the nonverbal context (given information). Greenfield and Smith (1976) state that in the one-word stage, "What, from the child's point of view, can be assumed is not stated; what cannot be taken for granted is given verbal expression" (p. 186). They cite several examples of this principle. In an agent-action relationship, children at the one-word stage usually take the agent for granted but find the action or change of state to be less certain. Therefore they choose to encode the action or state rather than the agent. For example, in referring to daddy running, the child likely would say "run" rather than "daddy." To refer to their dirty hand, children would say "dirty" rather than "hand." If the condition to be verbalized is a relation between an action or state and its object, children encode the action or state in one circumstance and the object in another. In general, they express the action or state if they hold the object in their possession as it is undergoing change. For example, if they are holding a paper that is tearing, they would say "tear." If they are not in immediate possession of the object, they perceive it with less certainty and therefore encode the object. For example, if someone else broke a cup, the child would say "cup." Greenfield and Smith found similar choices in children's one-word answers to questions. They report that the children's verbal responses consisted of the most informative element in what would be considered an adult response form. Wells (1974), like Greenfield and Smith, indicates that children choose to express the information that they perceive to be most essential for the listener to interpret what they say. Similarly, Brown (1973) reports that in Stage I of development (MLU 1.0–2.0), children tend to omit words whose meanings can be recognized on the basis of nonlinguistic context. Bates (1976) and Greenfield and Smith (1976) propose that the child's early differentiation of new and given information is the initial step in learning the proposition-presupposition relationship expressed later in more mature language forms.

Children's early choice of words for expression may be based more on their efforts to resolve their own uncertainty than on their recognition of what may be unknown to their listener. In other words, children may select for encoding the word that represents new information for them rather than what they perceive to be unknown to another person.

de Villiers and de Villiers (1978) propose certain skills which children must have in order to be able to modify their speech according to the situation and their relationship with the listener. They suggest that the child must have:

1. Enough flexibility of grammar and vocabulary to be able to choose among speech codes.
2. A recognition that different listeners have different needs in conversation; for example, that a stranger will need more explicit information than a close family member.
3. A recognition that certain modes of address are more polite than others.
4. The ability to tell which audience deserves, or will demand, a more polite or formal style. (de Villiers and de Villiers 1978, p. 163)

At age 2, children show little recognition of what information the listener needs or has regarding the topic of conversation. While adults rarely center their statements around information the listener has, children frequently tell adults things that they are already aware of (Bloom and Lahey 1978). This is seen in the young child's comments about visible activities and items in the immediate environment. At age two, children seem incapable of or uninterested in selecting content and form on the basis of the listener's needs.

Between three and four years of age, children begin to make assumptions about listeners' access to information relative to the topic of discussion. Maratsos (1973) found that children of this age provide more detailed information when describing toys to a listener they believe to be blind than when giving such descriptions to persons they consider to have normal vision. This suggests that children in the three to four year age range have learned to make judgments about the listener's needs and to adapt the content of their verbalizations according to what they perceive to be the listener's prior or shared knowledge.

Shatz and Gelman (1978) found that four-year-old children use different form and content when talking to two year olds than when talking to another four year old or to an adult. When addressing two year olds, they expressed simpler content and used more direct forms to control the younger child's attention. Shatz and Gelman noted that the four year olds seemed to select linguistic forms that resulted in the least ambiguity possible. They state that the alterations made in talking to younger children result from the speaker's perceptions of the child's level of cognitive, social, and linguistic maturity. de Villiers and de Villiers (1978), agreeing with Shatz and Gelman, state that by age four, children have become more aware of the listener's prior knowledge and abilities and have begun learning to encode more clearly new as opposed to old information. They report that by age five, children show even greater modifications in utterance content and form to accommodate the listener's needs and capabilities.

Children learn to adjust their utterances not only to provide necessary information to listeners but also to suit their social role and status relationship with the listener. Berko-Gleason (1973) notes that young children first show social adaptations by choosing to vocalize or not to vocalize in a particular context. In the early stages of speech, it is not uncommon for a child to vocalize freely or to say some familiar phrase such as *bye-bye* in the presence of family members but to refuse to vocalize when strangers are present. The ability to alter linguistic form according to the child's perceptions of social relationships is not seen until a child is about three years of age (Bloom and Lahey 1978). Bates (1976) reports that between three and one half and four years of age, children begin to use indirect rather than direct forms of requests, thus demonstrating a sensitivity to the context as well as the ability to change linguistic form to conform to social conventions. She states that children do not substitute more polite forms (*I would like—*——) for previously used direct forms (*Gimme a*———) until four and one half to five years of age. Garvey (1975) notes that five year olds use twice as many indirect request forms as three year olds, while the two groups use about the same number of direct request forms. Garvey (1975) and Shatz and Gelman (1978) report that while children three years old and younger respond appropriately to adults' indirect requests for action, it is likely that their responses are based on an interpretation of the core meaning of the proposition in light of the immediate nonverbal context rather than on a recognition of the underlying linguistic structure of indirect requests.

Presuppositions: Examples of Disordered Development

Children who do not learn to recognize another person's perspective and adapt what they say accordingly are not successful in conversation. They may not understand the meaning of what someone says when shared but unspoken information provides a frame of reference for interpreting the statement. This may result from the child's failure to integrate another person's statement with the nonverbal context. A problem of this nature is evidenced in the following interchange between a teacher and a child as they watched another child fall from a bicycle and cut his arm:

Teacher: Uh-oh. We need to get a band-aid.
Child: What for?

The child's response suggested that she did not recognize the presupposed commonality of reference provided by the shared nonverbal information.

Some children with language disorders do not relate specific utterances to what has been said in a previous utterance. A problem of this nature is apparent in the following exchange:

Clinician (reading a story to the child): Bill pushed Tommy off the swing. Tommy ran into the house crying.
Child: Why was Tommy crying?

Further experiences in conversing with the children in these two examples indicated that they frequently interpreted what was said as though each utterance should stand alone. They often experienced confusion in meaning when they had to recognize the underlying presuppositions upon which an utterance was based.

Some children with language disorders either presuppose too much or disregard the listener's prior knowledge so that the listener has difficulty recognizing the frame of reference to which the child's comments apply. When talking with children with problems of this nature, adults may feel that they have entered a conversation in the middle or that they were not paying attention when the child indicated to what his or her statement refers. The following incident reflects such a difficulty:

> Five-year-old Ray walked into a clinician's office and said, "She didn't want me to do that anymore." The clinician asked a number of questions before determining that the child was attempting to tell her that he had thrown a toy car through a window at school that morning and his teacher did not want him to do that again.

A similar problem was indicated by an incident reported by the mother of a four-year-old child with disordered language:

> Carrie came out of her room and announced to her mother, "Julie didn't give me that book." Not knowing anyone named Julie or what book the child was referring to, the mother was unable to make sense of the statement. The mother's questioning finally brought out that Julie was a child in Carrie's nursery school and that Julie had refused to give Carrie a particular book the previous day.

Both of these children were unable to participate successfully in conversation because they did not know how to determine what was new and what was shared information; they did not know how to adapt what they said so that they enjoyed a common point of reference with the addressee.

Language-disordered children may not alter what they say or how they say it according to their social roles relative to the listener or to meet the demands of a social situation They may not use indirect forms of request or polite forms in communication with other people. The report of the parent of a five year old is illustrative:

> "Karen never tries to get her way by being sweet," complained Karen's mother. The mother contrasted her daughter's indiscriminate use of "Gimme that" or "Stop it" with her peers' use of "May I have that?" or "I don't want you to do that." Karen's mother recognized that her child's ineffectiveness in communicating often resulted from a failure to adapt her means of expression according to the social context.

Children who do not alter what they say and how they say it may not recognize that they would be more effective if their utterances were more socially appropriate, or they may not have the linguistic skills to alter the way they phrase their utterances. Some may not recognize the social indicators on which mature speakers depend for guidance in formulating utterances to meet social demands.

Language-disordered children's presuppositional abilities have been the study of a limited amount of research. Snyder (1975, 1978) found that language-disordered children who used primarily single-word utterances encoded less-informative elements almost as often as they encoded more-informative elements in the conversational situation. Their peers with normal language usually encoded the most informative elements. In a study of older preschool children with language disorders, Fey, Leonard, and Wilcox (1980) investigated the children's alterations in verbalizations directed to younger children compared with their verbalizations directed to their age peers. They found that when addressing the younger children, the language-disordered children reduced the mean preverb length, used internal state questions more frequently, and seemed to be more conversationally assertive. From this study, it seems that some language-disordered children can and do alter what they say and how they say it according to their listener.

Deixis Rees (1978) explains, "Deixis is the term for linguistic devices that anchor the utterance to the communicative setting in which it occurs"(p. 210). In conversation we use linguistic expressions to indicate persons who are and are not participating in the conversation, locations relative to the speaker, and time of occurrence relative to the time of conversation. Clark and Sengul (1978) comment, "Deictic terms 'point to' places, times, or participants in a conversation—from the speaker's point of view"(p. 461).

In English, personal pronouns are the primary deictic terms for *person*. The speaker is referred to by first person pronouns; the listener by second person pronouns; and others by common nouns, proper nouns, or third person pronouns. Deictic expressions of *place* refer to the location of events or entities referred to in the conversation relative to the location of the speaker. Terms such as *this, that, here, there, come, go, bring,* and *take* are elements of the place deictic system. Linguistic devices indicating *time* mark events or conditions referred to as present, past, or future relative to the moment of conversation. Deictic expressions for time include tense markers for verbs as well as lexical items such as *yesterday, later, recently,* and *tomorrow*.

Linguistic deixis is a discourse phenomenon. It expresses the relationship between a referent and the occasion of the utterance. Deixis can be learned only through language use in communicative interactions. In the person, place, and time deictic systems, the speakers' perspective is the central point from which reference is made. Proximal/distal distinctions relative to the speaker are basic in all three categories.

In order to understand and to use deictic expressions, persons must recognize that these terms have a point of reference, that they involve reference shifting, and that at times they have shifting reference boundaries (Clark and Sengul 1978). One must be able to exchange roles, to recognize another's perspective, in order to learn deixis.

Deixis: Normal Development

Bruner (1975, 1978) reports that in infant-caregiver prelinguistic interactions, infants learn to follow another's line of regard, to signal line of focus, and to reverse roles in give-and-take play routines. He states that "... these accomplishments guarantee the first bases for spatial, interpersonal deixis" (Bruner 1978, p. 31). Clark and Sengul (1978) report that the frequency of shift in reference point influences the order of acquisition of personal pronouns. *I* always refers to the person speaking and only shifts referent when the speaker changes. *You* shifts not only when the speaker changes but also when the speaker addresses a different listener. Third person pronoun referents change more frequently than those for *I* or *you*. They are different each time the speaker refers to a different third party. Clark and Sengul (1978) consider that the order of acquisition of personal pronouns (*I* before *you*; *you* before *he* and *she*) can be accounted for by the relative frequency of change in referents for each. Similarly, the de Villiers (1978) contend that person deictic terms are learned more easily than expressions of place because they have a fixed reference point, requiring a change from the speaker's to the listener's perspective but not an understanding of relative distance.

As with person deixis, the order in which deictic expressions of place are learned is influenced by the number or frequency of shifts in referents associated with them (de Villiers and de Villiers 1978; Clark and Sengul 1978). For example, fewer shifts are required in using proximal terms (*here, this, these*), which always mean near the speaker, than in using distal terms (*there, that, those*), which can refer to any place except the immediate proximity of the speaker. From this theory, it is predictable that *here* and *this* will be learned before *there* and *that*. Clark and Sengul (1978) report that most children first use themselves as the point of reference for interpreting place deictic terms, although a lesser percentage may use the speaker as the reference point from the beginning. Charney (1979) concludes that children are more likely to experience confusion in understanding *here* and *there* if the speaker's use of the terms requires an orientation directly opposite the child's.

Terms that adults use to express deixis of place appear early in child language. Clark and Sengul (1978) note that the appearance of words such as *here, there, this,* and *that* does not mean that the child is using them in a deictic sense. To illustrate the nondeictic use of such terms, they report that children may use *here* to select objects and *there* to indicate that they have completed a task. Brown (1973) suggests that in stage I, children use *here* and *there* as prolocatives or as the names of places, seemingly without the proximal/distal contrast employed in the adult deictic system. Clark and Sengul (1978) report that as late as four years of age, children do not use *here/there* or *this/that* as true deictic contrasts. Clark and Garnica (1974) note that at two years of age, children use *come* and *go* as nondeictic verbs, but they do not use *come/go* and *bring/take* as deictic contrasts until after seven years of age.

Deixis of time is not learned until relatively late in the language-learning period, since young children speak about the present and have little need to mark past or future time. Brown (1973) observes that no tense markers are used in Stage I of language development. Generally, Brown's subjects did not use grammatical morphemes to signal time other than present until Stage III, which occurred around the third birthday for most children. Umiker-Sebeok (1979) reports that in children's spontaneous narratives, almost all narratives of three year olds pertained to events which took place in the immediate setting very near the time they were reported. In addition, children in this age group did not indicate linguistically the temporal orientation of the events about which they spoke. For four and five year olds, about half of the narratives pertained to prior events within the classroom and half to outside events. Both of the older age groups used linguistic devices to orient the events in their narratives with respect to time.

Deixis: Examples of Disordered Development

Children who do not learn to view themselves and other people as separate and to contrast their own with another person's perspective or viewpoint will not learn linguistic deixis. Experiences in role reversal are a prelude to deixis of person, place, and time. Failure to engage in alternate and reciprocal routines, either verbal or nonverbal, may indicate that children are not acquiring patterns of interaction which provide a framework for learning to use deictic terms. Some children do not produce or respond to nonlinguistic signals indicating line of regard. They may not point or look toward the item of their interest in an attempt to signal their line of attention, and they may not recognize the intentions of others' use of such gestures for this purpose. Until children learn the meaning of nonlinguistic forms indicating line of regard, they will not learn linguistic devices to orient the conversation with respect to person, place, and time.

Some children manifest deficits in using the system of person deixis. They may continue to use proper names rather than personal pronouns to refer to themselves and their partners in conversation. The following conversation between Jack, a five-year-old boy with disordered language, and his normally developing three-year-old sister, Paula, illustrates Jack's inappropriate use of proper names in referring to the person to whom he was speaking:

> *Paula:* I want some gum (reaching toward Jack, who was unwrapping a piece of gum).
> *Jack:* Paula can't have any of this gum (hiding the gum behind his back).

> *Paula:* I want some. You share!
>
> *Jack:* Paula get gum from Mommy. Mommy has Paula's gum. Paula can't have this (stuffing the gum into his mouth).

Personal pronouns may appear in the speech of some language-disordered children without being used as deictic contrasts. The following example illustrates the behavior of one language-disordered child who does not use person deictic terms appropriately:

> Jerry, a four year old with limited interactional speech or nonspeech behavior, used *she* to refer to people whose proper names he did not know. He used no other pronoun forms to refer to animate beings. Occasionally he used *it* with reference to inanimate objects (*Broke it* or *It's gone*) and as semantically empty forms with ambient verbs (*It's cold* or *It's raining*). To ask a person to open a jar for him, Jerry said, "Pat can open the jar," handing a jar to Pat, whose name he knew. To a new boy in the class, Jerry said, "She can wind up a dog," requesting that the classmate wind up a mechanical dog. In looking at a scratch on a boy's leg, Jerry commented, "She hurt the knee."

For Jerry, *she* appears as a general term referring to any person whose name he does not know. He uses *she* to refer to persons whom he is addressing as well as those about whom he is speaking. He does not use this term in the deictic sense in which it normally is used in adult language.

Misuse of deictic terms may interfere with the listener's interpretation of the speaker's intent. The following example illustrates such an instance:

> Ann, age five, interrupted an activity on the opening day of class by saying to the clinician, "My name is. . . ." The clinician responded, "Your name is Ann." Ann again said, "My name is. . . ." and the clinician again responded, "Your name is Ann." This exchange was repeated several times, with Ann's statement becoming more emphatic with each turn. In obvious exasperation, Ann then pointed to her classmate Tommy and said, "My name is Tommy," to Leslie and said, "My name is Leslie," and then looked toward the clinician and said, "My name is. . . ." Finally recognizing Ann's intentions, the clinician stated her own name. Ann nodded and returned to her previous activity.

While Ann ultimately came up with a way to get her point across to the person whom she was addressing, her inappropriate use of *my* was confusing to the clinician and resulted in a misinterpretation of Ann's intent.

Pronoun reversal frequently is cited as a characteristic of speech of autistic children (Baltaxe and Simmons 1975; Fay and Schuler 1980). Their failure to make you/I distinctions in verbal interactions may be evidence of a deficit in learning the linguistic system of deixis or may result from failure to acquire the prerequisite ability to contrast their own with another person's point of view.

While linguistic deixis of place is learned only to a limited extent in the preschool years, certain patterns of language acquisition suggest that particular children are not gaining the language skills prerequisite to mastery of place deixis. Those who are not learning person deixis are likely to have difficulties with place deixis. Deficits in learning the linguistic system for deixis of place can be predicted for children who do not make reference to locations of objects and events relative to another person and to themselves. A five year old with disordered language showed such a pattern of language use:

> Ted, age five, made reference linguistically to the static location of objects and people. He used utterances such as *Baby (is) on the table* and *Blocks (are) in the box* appropriately in describing the locations of objects. Ted did not encode locative relations referring to directional movement (*He went to the store*) or locations defined by relative distance from himself or another person (*Stand by me* or *Sit close to the teacher*). The locations which he encoded linguistically (usually referring to containment) were those which would be the same from anyone's perspective. He did not use linguistic devices whose meanings were dependent on the spatial orientation of different people.

Predictably, Ted did not use place deictic terms in a contrastive sense. Before learning the linguistic system for deixis of place, he had to learn to refer linguistically to locations relative to different people and to those defined by relative distance, both from himself and from other people.

Children with language disorders often show evidence of deficits in learning linguistic deixis of time. Perhaps the most frequently noted indication of such deficits is the failure to use past tense verb forms to indicate time of occurrence of a reported event relative to the occasion of its reporting. The following conversation between five-year-old Billy and a clinician illustrates this type of problem:

> *Billy:* Last night my brother kick me.
>
> *Clinician:* Why did he kick you?
> *Billy:* I break his truck.
>
> *Clinician:* What happened when he kicked you?
> *Billy:* I cry. I tell daddy and daddy spank him.

Billy used lexical items (*last night*) to mark the time of the event he reported, but he did not alter verb forms to signal prior occurrence. Some children with language disorders may not even use lexical items to orient the content of their utterances with respect to time, leaving their listeners confused about the temporality of reported events. Terms such as *yesterday, next time, tommorow,* and *later* may not be used to establish time relative to the present.

Children with language disorders may restrict their comments to the here-and-now, referring only to events within the immediate context. Until they begin to make reference to or to report on occasions other than the present, they have no need for linguistic devices to orient the content of their utterances with respect to time. Analysis of their language will show an absence of time deictic markers, but this may reflect cognitive or language deficits other than a failure to learn the linguistic system for time deixis.

summary of pragmatics

From an early age, children act with the intent of accomplishing certain purposes. Their prelinguistic and then linguistic communicative behaviors can be described according to the functions served or the intended effects. Consideration of the purposes for which children use language provides a means for describing the efficiency and effectiveness with which they communicate. Some language-disordered children use language for a limited range of purposes. Their language does not serve them in all the ways it serves normally developing children. The restrictions in communicative intents expressed by some children with deviant language may result in a lack of need or motivation to learn language. Failures to learn to encode certain intents linguistically may reduce their effectiveness in interpersonal communication and in exploring their world.

Learning to use language in conversation is important in order for children to put language to full use. Around age three, normally developing children show an increased understanding of conversational rules and of procedures which enhance the flow of conversation. They learn to adapt what they say and how they say it to meet listeners' needs and to conform to the demands of the social context. They learn linguistic devices to orient the content of their utterances with respect to persons, place, and time. Children with language disorders may be deficient in conversational abilities and therefore find it difficult to engage in dialogue. Inadequate conversational skills result in their misinterpretation of what others say and in others' misinterpretation of what they say. Those who cannot be successful in conversation will be restricted severely in their effective use of language.

○ SEMANTICS

The semantic component of language is "...the linguistic representation of what persons know about the world of objects, events, and relations" (Bloom and Lahey 1978, p. 14). It is the content of language and can be described in terms of *referential* and *propositional* meanings. Words that denote people, objects, actions and processes, conditions, ideas, and attributes comprise the referential component. In early child language, these words usually make reference to observable entities, actions, and attributes, and are classified grammatically as nouns, verbs, and adjectives. Other words mark grammatical structures, semantic relations, and carry more subtle meanings. In traditional grammar, they are classified as auxiliary or copular verbs, articles, prepositions, and conjunctions. Brown (1973) states that such words, along with inflections on nouns and verbs, modulate the major meanings of sentences, and he classifies them as grammatical morphemes. In the present discussion, the learning of grammatical morphemes will be a part of the discussion of syntax.

Propositional meanings are the predications or assertions put forth in utterances. Propositions go beyond the referential meanings of individual lexical items. They are compositional meanings, identified by the semantic relations between the verb and noun elements in an utterance. The present discussion will include both referential and propositional meanings as components of the content of children's utterances.

referential meanings of words

A word is used to denote a category of actions, states, objects, and so on. Concepts represented by words are defined by semantic features that determine which experiences are referred to appropriately by one word and which should be represented by a different word. There is a point at which the word *chair* is not appropriate and *couch* is chosen, when *pretty* replaced by *beautiful,* when *run* is used rather than *walk,* when *ecstatic* fits better than *happy,* and when *blue* becomes *green.* If language is to function as a device which people use to share information or meanings, the language users must assign similar boundaries to the concepts to which words refer.

Clark (1973) states that "... the meanings of words can be broken down into some combination of units of meaning smaller than that represented by the word" (p.74). In her Semantic Feature Hypothesis, Clark proposes that the meaning of a word is composed of critical features that delimit the categories of experience to which the word applies. For example, the critical features for *woman* include /+human/, /+female/, /+adult/, while those for girl would include /+human/, /+female/, and /–adult/. In learning the meaning of a word, a child must determine which combination of semantic features define the category to which that word applies.

Knowing a word includes recognizing its referent, both in a particular instance and across a variety of conditions (Bloom and Lahey 1978). One needs to know that the word *table* may refer to a certain table in one's home as well as to a class of objects which share similar features but may vary within limits in size, shape, and composition. Knowledge of the word *kick* requires recognition that it refers not only to what people do when their foot strikes a ball, but also to what a horse does when it rears its hind legs and to what people do with their legs when swimming. The range of conditions to which a word can apply determines its use.

Knowledge of a word includes knowing that the referent is part of a more general category of experiences that have certain aspects of meaning in common. Anglin (1977) explains that words are organized according to features of meaning that fit into hierarchical relations. Figure 2–2 illustrates the hierarchical relationships between particular instances of entities and their more generic classes. Anglin points out that such hierarchical relations facilitate organization of information as well as memory. Recognizing the characteristics which lead to categorization at any point in the hierarchy requires one to integrate information about an array of objects and experiences.

Just as words referring to objects can be grouped into semantic categories, verbs too can be subdivided on the basis of shared aspects of meaning. Chafe (1970) identifies five verb types which are defined by semantic properties. Verbs which state an action and require the accompaniment of a stated or implied initiator of the action are called *action* verbs. These include words such as *run* and *sing*. *Process* verbs, such as *shrink* or *die*, specify a change in state or condition of a noun. *Action-process* verbs express both what an initiator of the action does and a change in state of an entity. *Kill* and *paint* are action-process verbs. *State* verbs identify a particular condition of a noun or verb. *Broken, dead,* and *happy* are examples of states. In traditional grammar, states of nouns generally are classified as adjectives, predicate nouns, prepositional phrases, clauses, or verbs. Chafe identifies a fifth verb type, *ambient,* which can stand alone as a predication without having an accompanying semantically related noun. Ambient verbs are predications which are all-encompassing states or events and are ". . . without reference to some particular 'thing' within the environment" (Chafe 1970, p 102). For

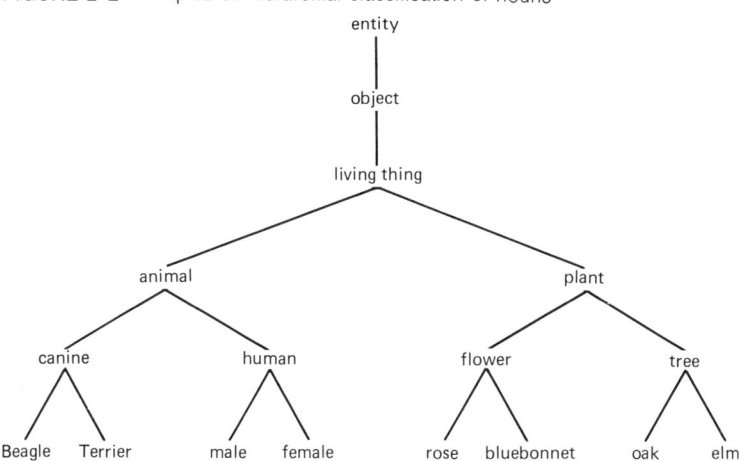

FIGURE 2–2 Examples of Hierarchial classification of nouns

```
                        entity
                          |
                        object
                          |
                     living thing
                     /           \
                animal            plant
               /      \          /     \
           canine    human    flower    tree
           /  \      /  \     /    \    /  \
       Beagle Terrier male female rose bluebonnet oak elm
```

example, in the sentences *It's late* and *It's snowing, late* identifies a state and *snowing* refers to an action, both covering the environment but not tied semantically to a particular entity.

Words designating attributes can be subclassified according to the nature of their meanings. Some words refer to characteristics which contrast one object with another, thus denoting an identifying feature of a particular entity. Other words make reference to a change in condition or a transitory state of an object. For example, *red* may be a constant feature of a particular cup, while *broken* refers to an alteration in the condition of the cup. de Villiers and de Villiers (1978) point out that appropriate use of certain words designating attributes of objects requires comparisons to a standard of reference that changes from object to object and from context to context. For example, *big* as a description of a child's toy bus is based on a different size standard than when it is used to describe the city bus on which persons ride to work. The standard used when describing a downtown building as *little* is different from the standard by which an animal or a person is judged as *little*. Appropriate use of such words requires recognition of relevant properties and shifting standards of reference.

In learning to use words referentially, children show certain patterns of development as they move from the limited meanings they first assign to words to the definitions shared by adult speakers of a language. Recognition of these patterns of learning sheds light on some of the factors which influence children's learning of word meanings. It also assists in determining whether a child is learning to use words referentially in a normal manner and provides guidance in planning and carrying out remediation programs for children who are not learning language normally.

Referential Meanings: Normal development Children and adults who talk to them are active participants in the word-learning process. Among the factors that appear to influence which words children learn first as well as their patterns of learning word meanings are:

1. The child's own experiences
2. Actions and changes in the environment
3. The communicative functions words serve
4. The context in which language is used
5. Parental patterns of language use and their responsiveness to the child's verbal attempts.

Consideration of these factors may provide insight into the word-learning process.

Children's own experiences influence their choice of words to learn and patterns of learning. Their early words refer to persons and objects with which they have direct contact and to events in which they are involved. Nelson (1977) contends that children establish the core meaning of a concept or category to which object words refer through their manipulations of items and not through passive observation. Children's earliest verbs refer to actions they initiate or are affected by and to changes in objects they manipulate. Their direct interactions with their environment determine what words they learn as well as the meanings they assign to lexical items.

Children's early words usually are associated with *actions and changes in their environment.* They show an interest in words referring to entities that act, are acted upon, or change states (Nelson 1973, 1974; Huttenlocher 1974; Anglin 1977). Words expressing action events (*run, eat*) appear in children's speech before those encoding experiential states (*see, want*). Bloom, Lightbrown, and Hood (1975) found that children first learn verbs that encode movements affecting only the actor (*run, jump*), those in which the actor brings about a movement of another object (*ride, open*), and those resulting in a change in location of an object (*throw, put*). Wells (1974) reports that verbs referring to changes in physical conditions of objects (*cut, break*) appear early in child language. Children's first words designating properties, conditions, or attributes of objects usually refer to changeable or transitory states (*wet, broken, dirty*) rather than to permanent conditions of objects (*big, round, red*) (Wells 1974; Bowerman 1976). The de Villiers (1978) note that children initially are attuned to changing or atypical conditions of objects with which they interact and therefore show an interest in learning words that represent such phenomena.

The *communicative functions words serve* for a child influences which words he or she learns first. Nelson (1973) found that some children show an early preference for words that label objects in their surroundings. These children, referred to by Nelson as *Referential,* most often use words to direct attention to or to label objects. Other children's early words generally encode some type of interpersonal interaction. Nelson calls these children *Expressive* and states that they show a greater interest in learning words to regulate social interactions. She points out that the distinction between children who use words to label and those who use words in a social, regulatory sense is not dichotomous but rather occurs on a continuum. As children learn to express the variety of communicative intents described earlier in the discussion of the pragmatics of child language, they are motivated to learn the meaning of lexical items that will increase the effectiveness of their communicative efforts. In this way, learning to encode new pragmatic intentions encourages expansion in knowledge of word meanings.

de Villiers and de Villiers (1978) illustrate the effect of communicative need on children's learning of words referring to static states or attributes. They explain that children learn words to refer to static states only when they have a need to subclassify a category of objects or to designate one out of a group of similar items. When they realize that their intents will be interpreted more accurately if they use words that contrast certain items or actions with others in a common class, they learn words that specify the particular one to which they are referring. For example, at this point, children contrast *red ball* with *green ball* and *big cookie* with *little cookie* because such contrasts serve an important purpose for them.

The *context in which language is used* has an impact on children's learning of word meanings. In early stages of language learning, most speech directed to the child refers to the here-and-now, and often it is accompanied by relevant actions or gestures from the speaker. Young children rely heavily on the nonlinguistic context for clues to the meaning of what is said. With increasing facility they use the linguistic context to assist them in learning word meanings. By three to four years of age, they gain information about a word's grammatical class and thus clues to its meaning from its grammatical role in sentences (Brown 1958). They also draw conclusions about semantic properties of objects and actions to which a word refers from the verbal context (de Villiers and de Villiers 1978). Once they know that a verb such as *jump* refers to an action initiated by an animate being, they can conclude that the agent (or subject) of this verb has the feature /+ animate/, even if they do not know the meaning of the word designating the one who jumped. If children hear the sentence "The aardvark jumped up and hurt its front legs," they might conclude that an aardvark not only has the feature /+ animate/ but also has the feature /-human/, since humans do not have front legs. In this manner, children learn to discover meanings of words through their occurrence in certain verbal contexts.

Parental patterns of language use and responsiveness to the child's verbal attempts have an influence on children's learning of words. Nelson (1973) indicates that mothers who emphasize labels for objects and their properties when talking to their young children are likely to have children who at first show a preference for learning words which serve a naming function. Mothers who most often use language to direct their young children's activities tend to have children whose major interest is in words that express some aspect of social interaction.

Brown (1967) discusses the partnership role of children and adults in the word-learning process. He states that children hear an adult use a word in the presence of certain items or events and then use the word under similar circumstances. They rely on feedback from mature speakers to determine whether the meaning they have assigned to the word coincides with the adult's usage. Referring to the child as the "player" and the mature speaker as the "tutor" in the word-learning process, Brown states:

> In simple concrete terms the tutor says "dog" whenever a dog appears. The player notes the equivalence of these utterances, forms a hypothesis about the nonlinguistic category that elicits this kind of utterance, and then tries naming a few dogs himself. (Brown 1967, p. 285)

If an adult responds in ways the child does not intend, the child is likely to modify his or her conclusions about the nonlinguistic categories to which words refer. Gradually through hypothesis testing and alterations motivated by the acceptability or effectiveness of their utterances, children learn the range of experiences to which a word applies in the adult version of their language. Parents' feedback to their children who are trying out new words has an impact on the children's learning of the meanings of words.

Developmental Patterns in Learning Word Meanings

To learn what words mean, children must figure out how words are used to represent the concepts they have formed, and, in certain instances, they must reorganize prelinguistic categories to fit the linguistic categories of their native language. Bowerman (1978b) states, "An important task for the child acquiring words is to determine the nature and boundaries of the categories or concepts to which they refer" (p. 361).

Children's early use of words generally does not mirror adult usage. The boundaries for the concepts to which they assign words may be more narrow or broader than those governing adults' definitions of words. Initially, children associate a word with a particular referent, which becomes the prototypical object, action, or state with which the word is associated (Anglin 1977; Bowerman 1978a; de Villiers and de Villiers 1978). Then they use the word with referents which share certain features with the prototypical exemplar. This results in overextension and underextension in word use. Overextensions are seen in young children's use of object labels as well as in their use of words referring to actions and attributes. They may use the word *dog* to refer to all four-legged animals, seemingly using this characteristic as a primary semantic feature that regulates the use of this word. Bowerman (1978a) reports that her daughter overextended use of the word *kick,* employing it not only to refer to her foot striking something but also to other actions which entailed movement of a limb (a moth flying) and sudden contact with a body part (bumping into an object). In reference to a table that was setting at an unusual angle rather than against the wall, a young child said to the author, "That table is wrinkled," providing an example of an overextension of an attributive word. Underextensions occur when children use a word to refer to a more restricted set of items than the word encompasses in adult language. Bloom (1973) cites the example of her daughter's use of the word *car* to refer only to cars which passed along the street as she watched from the window of her home. She did not use *car* to refer to cars in which she was riding, pictures of cars, or parked cars. Bowerman (1978a) states that her daughter underextended her use of the word *off.* She restricted use of this word to references to the removal of clothing or other objects from the body.

Children learning language normally often overextend and underextend the meanings of label and action words during their first year of speaking, usually between the ages of one and two and one-half years old. Clark (1973, 1974) indicates that overextensions demonstrate that the child's semantic categories are defined by general semantic features, such as four-leggedness, and do not yet include more specific defining characteristics. Bowerman (1976) suggests that underextensions reflect the child's association of the word with a more restricted set of features than adults assign to the word. Through their use of words in meaningful contexts and with feedback from adults, children restructure the conceptual categories to which they assign words so that they include the relevant semantic features that define the word as it is used by adults.

de Villiers and de Villiers (1978) discuss children's patterns of learning the meanings of words designating attributes of objects. They explain that learning certain words referring to attributes requires recognition of standards of reference that change with the context. *Big* and *little* are the first attributes of this nature to appear in children's speech. At two and three years of age, children generally use these words in an absolute sense, with their personal experiences as the standard of reference. By about four years, they begin to show a sensitivity to context and refer to objects as *big* or *little* in light of the situation in which they are used. The de Villiers cite an example of two-, three-, and four-year-old children who were playing tea party using a set of small toy people and a shot glass for the people to drink from. When asked if the glass was big or little, the younger children replied that it was little, apparently using their own size standard for glasses in making the judgment. The four year olds gave responses that indicated that the glass was big with reference to the toy people. One even stated that it was little by her own standards but big for the small toy people.

Many attributive words occur in antonymous pairs (*big/little; long/short; tall/short; wide/narrow*). Dimensional adjective pairs refer to polar extremes, with the positive term referring to the most extended aspect of the dimension and the negative term to the least extended. Some studies of children's acquisition of dimensional adjectives have indicated that children tend to use positive pole adjectives earlier and more frequently than their negative counterparts (Wales and Campbell 1970; Clark 1973). Greenfield and Smith (1976) suggest that young children do not necessarily learn positive before negative pole adjectives. They propose that a child learns one member of the polar pair in a specific context, and the member of the pair learned first is the one which refers to a change from the normal state of the object to which it is attributed. There is no evidence that children learn both members of polar pairs simultaneously. For a time, they are likely to contrast *big* with *not big* and *new* with *not new* rather than *big* with *little* and *new* with *old.*

Learning Words Representing Hierarchical Classifications

A part of learning the meaning of a word is recognizing that its referent is a member of a more general class of experiences and that there may be words that represent more specific instances of the general category to which a word refers. Children usually learn category labels that are at an intermediate level of generality before those that name object categories at the more specific or the more general level (Brown 1958; Anglin 1977; de Villiers and deVilliers 1978). Anglin (1977) observed that two- and three-year-old children used the word *flower* to refer to different types of plants, while some four and five year olds named the specific type of flower and used the more general term *plant.* The de Villiers (1978) point out that children learn appropriate use of a word more easily if the scope of application for the word corresponds with the child's categorization of objects on a perceptual and functional level. Brown (1958) and Anglin (1977) explain that in the life of a young child, needs are met through verbal reference at a midlevel of generality. For example, young children have little or no need to make reference to specific kinds of flowers or breeds of dogs, or for identifying more generic classes such as animals or plants. Therefore they are likely to learn the word *flower* before *rose* or *violet,* and before *plant.* They probably will use *dog* prior to *beagle, terrier,* or *bulldog,* and before *animal.* Brown and Anglin note that parents seem to realize that children's communicative needs are served best by words at an intermediate level of generality. In speaking to their children, they tend to use words at a midlevel of generality and gradually refer to more general and more specific levels as the child advances in age and language abilities.

Children's learning of dimensional adjectives, as explained by de Villiers and de Villiers (1978), follows a pattern similar to that seen in their learning of object and action labels at varying levels of generality and specificity. Children usually learn the dimensional adjectives *big* and *little,* which refer to general size, before the names for specific dimensions such as length or height (Clark 1973, 1977). Children as old as four and five years describe specific dimensions of length, width, and height with the words *big* and *little. Tall* and *short* as well as *long* and *short* generally are learned next, followed by *wide* and *narrow* and then *thick* and *thin* (de Villiers and de Villiers 1978). Clark (1977) claims that this order of acquisition occurs because words that refer to more specific dimensions have more constraints on their usage and therefore are more complex than words that apply to several dimensions.

Referential Meanings: Examples of Disordered Development
Children with language disorders may fail to learn words to refer to entities, events, and conditions in their world. In some cases, they seem unaware that

verbal symbols stand for specific parts of their nonverbal experiences so that they neither understand words used by someone else nor use words to represent people, objects, actions, or states. Children may use words as performatives but not in a referential sense when communicating with other people. Such children seem to use language in a pragmatic sense, that is, to serve certain performative functions, but they have difficulty using language to represent content. Children with this pattern of language development may use many terms such as *hi, please, no,* and *uh-oh,* yet fail to use words that stand for items, actions, or attributes.

Some children with language disorders learn to express certain types of concepts through words, but their lexicon does not include items representing other types of concepts. They may learn words referring to tangible items (*book, milk, doll*) but not to actions (*run, jump*), processes (*eat, break*), or states (*big, green*). A child may learn words to refer to some specific items but continue to use these words as though they were proper nouns rather than to represent categories of similar entities. Such a child will use a word in a context-specific manner, and at times an item-specific manner, rather than generalizing its use to a broad class of experiences. For example, the child may use *cat* only with reference to her own pet. Another child may continue to use a word to represent a whole category of items that share some perceptual or functional features so that overgeneralization in word usage extends past the age at which it occurs normally. For example, a four-year-old child with disordered language used *mailman* to refer to a mailman, a mailbox, a mail truck, and letters or packages. Children like this may rely almost exclusively on either perceptual or functional properties in determining the meaning of words. They may use a particular word to refer to all items which act or are used similarly and not learn that different words denote subclasses of items within the broad category defined by a particular behavior or function. They may continue to use words based on classes determined by perceptual features, failing to differentiate items on the basis of their utility or behavior.

Some older preschool children continue to use words to represent categories at a midlevel of generalization but do not learn those that represent the more generic classes or the more specific categories of items. Some children in this age group do not seem to gain information about the meaning of a word from the verbal context in which it occurs. They appear to learn words representing entities or actions with which they have had direct experience and those they need to serve their own needs, but they do not learn words which relate to other people's experiences or which have not been required for them to accomplish their own purposes. Some older preschool children show difficulty in learning attributive words which require a shifting standard of reference. They continue to use these words with themselves as the standard of reference but fail to learn to use them relative to other people, objects, or events. Children with language-learning deficits may not learn to use words to contrast one item or person with another. They may use words representing static states only in a nominal sense, while their age peers and adults use such words in a contrastive manner.

Children with language disorders may not recognize that most phenomena which they encounter can be represented linguistically. Rather than learning words incidentally when they are exposed to them on a regular basis, they may learn only those words which are necessary for expressing something of immediate importance to them. During the first three years of life, children probably learn words which facilitate their organization and control of their immediate environment. Beyond that age, they learn to refer verbally to ideas, events, entities, feelings, and attributes that extend beyond their immediate activities. They learn words to represent experiences that other people have and to refer to less tangible phenomena. The author has observed that some children with language disorders show a breakdown in word learning at the point of learning words to represent other people's experiences or words that stand for abstract ideas or feelings. They only learn words to refer to items which they use personally, to stand for actions which they perform or wish to have performed, or to denote conditions or states which have some special significance for them. For these children, language continues to serve elementary functions, such as those suggested by Halliday in Phase I or Phase II. They do not attempt to use language in the more abstract sense described for Phase III, and therefore they have little need to learn words which would be necessary primarily at this level of language use.

propositional meanings

Prelinguistically, children learn that they and other beings initiate actions and that persons and objects may be affected as a result of actions. They attach meanings to changes in the conditions of their surroundings, noticing that things disappear and reappear as well as change states. They organize their environment spatially, becoming aware of the normal orientation of objects as well as the locations of events and entities. They recognize distinguishing attributes of people and objects and begin to associate particular things with certain people. This conceptual knowledge precedes children's being able to represent linguistically information about people objects, and events, and their relationships to each other.

In early speech, children learn to encode relational concepts they have formed prelinguistically through their interactions with the people and objects in their surroundings. Children's multiword utterances have compositional meanings which extend beyond the referential meanings of individual words. The compositional meanings can be described as semantic relations, similar in principle to those proposed by Fillmore (1968) and Chafe (1970).

Before using multiword utterances, children communicate relational concepts through single words used in conjunction with the nonlinguistic context (Greenfield and Smith 1976). Adults' interpretations of children's single-word utterances support the notion that they communicate content beyond the referential meanings of individual lexical items. For example, if a child extends his muddy hand and says "Dirty," the adult addressed will interpret the child's utterance as "My hand is dirty." If a child points to a toy car and says "Broke," the listener probably will interpret that utterance as "The car is broken." Greenfield and Smith (1976) present an extensive description of the combinatorial meanings expressed through children's single-word utterances and information available in the nonverbal context in which the word is spoken. They suggest that children's one-word utterances have an underlying propositional structure composed of the lexical item that is encoded plus the relevant nonlinguistic elements obvious in the immediate context. The term *holophrase* has been used to describe the use of a single word to express a proposition that an adult would encode in a whole sentence. This term implies that the child's single-word utterances stand for spoken propositions.

Brown (1973), Bloom (1973), and Dore (1975) argue against viewing the meaning of single-word utterances as linguistic representations of propositional meanings or semantic relations. Brown proposes that a child's use of single-word utterances in combination with the linguistic context to convey relational meanings suggests that the child has relational concepts but should not be interpreted to mean that this conceptual knowledge is linguistic in nature. Similarly, Bloom (1973) indicates that while children may use words which indicate they have certain relational concepts, their use of such words does not necessarily mean that they intend to express these concepts linguistically. Their one-word utterances may indicate certain conceptual knowledge but should not be interpreted as semantic knowledge beyond that expressed linguistically. Dore (1975) states that to view single-word utterances combined with nonlinguistic contextual clues as evidence of semantic knowledge is to confuse conceptual knowledge and linguistic knowledge. He recommends that a clear distinction be drawn "between knowledge of language and knowledge of the world" in order to "prevent basing claims about the former on data about the latter." (Dore 1975, p. 34) Dore presents a convincing argument that children's single-word utterances express pragmatic intentions in addition to the referential meanings of the individual lexical items. Like Brown and Bloom, he states that children should not be viewed as having semantic knowledge beyond that expressed linguistically.

In describing the semantic component of a child's language, whether for the purpose of investigating normal language acquisition or for assessing the communication abilities of a child with a language disorder, one must decide whether to attribute compositional meanings to single-word utterances or to require linguistic representation of relational concepts before crediting the child with expressing semantic relations. The author's biases are that one should attribute knowledge of semantic relations only to children who demonstrate knowledge of the linguistic representations of such notions. Children's use of single words in combination with nonlinguistic contextual clues may indicate their understanding of relational concepts and therefore a readiness to learn to express these concepts linguistically. However, only the linguistic expression of propositional content should be viewed as evidence that the child has this type of semantic knowledge.

Propositional Meanings: Normal Development Children, regardless of their native language, express a similar limited set of relational meanings when they begin combining words (Brown 1973; Bowerman 1973a,b, 1976). The concepts first expressed linguistically are the same conceptual relationships that the child acquired in the sensorimotor period just prior to the emergence of two-word utterances (Sinclair 1971; Brown 1973).

Children's earliest connected utterances generally include what Brown (1973) refers to as operations of reference, which are "the simple semantic set of nomination, recurrence, and nonexistence" (Brown 1973, p. 172). In nomination, the child calls attention to an object, using utterances such as *There dog* or *This book.* In the recurrence operation, the child comments on or requests the reappearance of a person, object, or action. Utterances such as *More cookie* or *Another baby* signal the child's awareness of or request for recurrence. Expressions of nonexistence request or comment on the absence of an entity and may include utterances such as *No more jump* or *Horsie all gone.* Negative statements of rejection and denial also appear in the early stages of two-word speech. Bloom and Lahey (1978) consider the operations of reference to be reflexive object relations, that is, to express "the relation of an object to itself or to an equivalent object from the same class" (Bloom and Lahey 1978, p. 109). Leonard (1976) reports that in general, operations of reference appear prior to the emergence of semantic relations that involve the relationship between people or objects and actions or processes, or between people, objects, and actions and their attributes or locations.

When children begin talking about relations between people, objects, and actions or processes, they most often talk about what they are doing or are going to do and what they want someone else to do (Bloom and Lahey 1978). Within a short time period, they begin expressing linguistically relational concepts involving what they see others doing, recognizing associations between people and objects, and identifying certain attributes of people, objects, and events.

In an analysis of the utterances of children speaking a number of different languages, Brown (1973) identified eight semantic relations which accounted for the majority of multiword utterances of children whose MLU was 1.0 to 2.0. Subsequent studies have supported Brown's findings. Figure

2-3, based on information from Fillmore (1968), Chafe (1970), and Brown (1973), provides definitions for each of the most frequently used semantic roles as well as those which were expressed less often by young children. Brown proposes that during this stage of language acquisition, children are learning to express a limited set of semantic relations, most frequently the following:

Agent and action: Mommy push. Baby stand up.
Action and object: Eat banana. Hit ball.
Agent and object: Boy (kick) ball. Brother (ride) bike.
Action and location: Jump (on the) bed. Run (on the) sidewalk.
Entity and location: Mommy (is in) kitchen. Book (is on) shelf.
Possessor and possession: Baby('s) hat. Cat('s) foot.
Entity and attribute: Red car. Cup broken.
Demonstrative and entity: There cookie. This doll.

FIGURE 2-3 Semantic Roles

Agent:	Someone or something that initiates an action. In young children's speech, the agent most often is an animate being.
Action:	A perceived movement.
Object:	A person or thing that changes state as a result of an action, or that receives the force of an action.
Location:	Reference to the juxtaposition of objects in space, to the goal of movements, or to the names of places.
Entity:	Any person or object with a distinct, separate existence.
Possessor:	One to whom something belongs.
Possession:	The entity that is possessed. In early speech, possessions are more often alienable than inalienable.
Attribute:	A characteristic of an entity which contrasts that entity with others in its class.
Demonstrative:	Words (often used in conjunction with pointing) to point out the presence of an entity.
Instrument:	An object which plays a role in bringing about a process or action but which is not the motivating force or instigator.
Beneficiary:	One who benefits, either positively or negatively, from the state, action, or process of the verb.
Experiencer:	One whose mental experience or mental processes are affected, or who is mentally disposed in some way.
Comitative:	An animate being involved in an action or process or in a state together with the agent or object.

Brown points out that while these eight semantic relations describe the majority of utterances of children whose MLU is from 1.0 to 2.0, others occur with lesser frequency. His observations included the infrequent appearance of expressions of instrument, beneficiary, experiencer, and comitative. Brown notes that certain other semantic relations which are a part of adult language were used by young children in a few utterances, but many of these seemed to be used in an idiosyncratic sense, probably being direct copies from a frequently heard phrase of a parent. Leonard (1976) reports that in general, children use relations involving actor, action, and object before those involving location, possession, and attribute, and that the use of experiencer and instrument relations are rare in the speech of children whose MLU does not exceed 2.0.

Studies of the relational meanings expressed by children indicate that the broad semantic categories, such as agent, location, and possessor, have more narrow definitions for young children than for adults. In the early stages of speech, agents generally are animate beings, even though this is not necessarily the case in adult language (Bowerman 1973a; Brown 1973). The young child is more likely to express *Mommy push* or *Sister hit* than *Ball roll* or *Car hit.* Bloom, Lightbrown, and Hood (1975) report that young children talk about locative relations that involve movement more frequently than they refer to static locations of objects. Children refer to objects that are moving toward or away from a place, specifying the goal of the movement, before they talk about the existing location of an object or event. This means that children use utterances referring to locative relations in action events, such as *Put block (on) table* or *Go outside,* before those identifying existing locations, such as *Daddy sitting chair* or *Book (on) table.* In expressing possessor-possession relations, children generally refer to alienable before inalienable possessions (Brown 1973). For example, relations such as *Baby('s) book* and *Mommy('s) purse* are likely to appear before *Daddy('s) nose* and *Dog('s) tail.* Bloom and Lahey (1978) state that children's early use of possessive forms indicates that the child associates a certain object with a particular person. They use terms such as *Baby('s) sock* to identify an object in terms of its association with someone. While this represents an introduction into the concept of possession, the broader concept which includes notions about personal ownership or obtaining and relinquishing property is not fully acquired until later. Attributive relations expressed in two- and three-word utterances are used in a nominal rather than a contrastive sense. In early speech, both attributive-entity and possessor-possession relations often are used to create new labels for objects, labels which are more specific than the general class name for the objects (Brown 1973; Bloom and Lahey 1978).

Brown (1973) describes a systematic pattern of expansion from two-word to longer utterances in terms of the semantic relations expressed. In moving from two-term to three-term or from three-term to four-term utterances, children either combine two sets of previously learned constituents or expand one so that the constituent itself becomes a relation. For example, if children have been expressing agent + action (*Jack throw*) and action + object (*throw rock*) utterances, they subsequently are likely to produce utterances which combine these units as agent + action + object (*Jack throw rock*). If they have been using two-term utterances, such as action + object (*hit ball*), they may expand the object into attribute + object (*big ball*), thereby producing a three-relation utterance (*Hit big ball*). Brown notes that the level of difficulty appears to be the same for three-term relations, whether they result from concatenation of three terms or from two terms with one term expanded. This conclusion is based on the observation that in children's speech, utterances of these two types emerge at approximately the same time. From his observations of the orderly progression in sentence expansion, Brown concludes that the number of semantic relations programmed into a single sentence is an indicator of the level of complexity of sentences.

Propositional Meanings: Examples of Disordered Development
Children's nonlinguistic expression of relational concepts, whether through gestures and other nonverbal demonstrations or through combining a single word with the nonlinguistic context, precedes their expressions of these relations linguistically. Their failure to encode relational meanings in linguistic form may indicate that they do not recognize that the combinatorial meanings of words represent their nonlinguistic relational concepts. Continued reliance on the nonlinguistic context and gestures used in conjunction with single words is evidence of a deficit in learning to encode semantic relations linguistically. The following description, given by the parent of a three year old, pictures a child who communicates relational concepts but does not represent them linguistically.

> Mrs. T. reported that Jay used many single words but no word combinations. She noted that he usually was able to make his point by combining single words with gestures, objects in the context, and noises associated with particular items or actions. To illustrate his success in communicating, she described his "reporting" of his accident on his tricycle. He pointed to the scratch on his elbow and then took his father into the yard, pointed to the tricycle, made a noise representing a crash, and then fell to the ground. In conjunction with his actions, he used the word *bike* when pointing to the tricycle and *uh-oh* when he fell to the ground. He used a similar pattern of gestures, pantomime, and single words to report his brother's pushing him down and to ask for a pencil to complete a drawing.

This child demonstrated knowledge of relational concepts and procedures for representing them, but he did not know how to express them linguistically.

Studies comparing language-disordered with normally developing children with respect to expression of semantic relations have indicated that the language-disordered group learn to express propositional meanings in the same order but at a slower rate than the group with normal language (Freedman and Carpenter 1976; Leonard, Bolders, and Miller 1976). When matched for MLU, there was no significant difference in the semantic relations expressed by the two groups, at least in the early stages of development.

Some children with deficient language may program two or three but no more semantic relations into a single utterance. They may not have learned a systematic procedure for expanding their utterances through concatenation or expansion of roles expressed in simpler utterances. Their verbalizations may be characterized by the use of a series of two-relation or three-relation utterances over an extended time period rather than by progression to more complex levels of utterances containing a greater number of relations. The following exchange between a four-year-old child with disordered language and his teacher illustrates the child's use of a series of simple utterances to make a point that could have been communicated in a single utterance containing a greater number of semantic relations:

> *Child:* Me kick. Kick ball. Big ball.
> *Teacher:* You kicked the big ball?
> *Child*
> *(nodding):* Kick ball. Big ball.

This child expressed semantic relations in two-term utterances but did not combine them into more complex three- or four-term utterances.

Children who use language to serve a limited number of functions may find little need to learn to encode certain relational concepts which are needed primarily to signal intents they do not express. For example, if they use language only to obtain some object or service, they may not have cause to express relations such as agent + action, since the performer of the action is of little consequence. If their major use of language is to bring someone into a social interaction, they may rarely find need to express entity + attribute or action + object, since these relational concepts are not vital to expression of their intents. Some children whose language deficits include limitations in expressing propositional meanings appear to have more basic deficiencies in learning to express a variety of intents.

For children with deficiencies in language content, language intervention programs can be planned and carried out in a manner that emphasizes this aspect of language. Children can learn to encode relational concepts in order to convey their specific intents with regard to particular people, objects, and events. Learning language form is an important aspect of learning to express relational concepts so that listeners will interpret intended meanings appropriately.

summary of semantics

Children learn to use language to represent their concepts about the world. They employ words to refer to items, people, processes, actions, and states or conditions. Subsequently, they learn to express relational notions so that their utterances encode propositions. Their learning of word meanings initially is influenced most heavily by their own actions and interactions with people and objects in their environment. Through hearing and using language in interactions with others, they learn what conceptual categories are represented by words in adult language usage. The relational concepts they first express represent concepts they have formed prelinguistically. With cognitive growth, the propositions they encode expand in number and complexity.

A failure to learn the semantic aspects of language interferes significantly with communication effectiveness. Many children with disordered language either do not learn the referential meanings of words, or they have difficulty encoding relational concepts linguistically. For children with deficits in the semantic aspects of language, intervention programs must include teaching them to employ language to represent their conceptual knowledge.

○ SYNTAX

Learning to use linguistic structures to represent various aspects of meaning is a major achievement of normally developing preschool children. The use of single words to represent certain elements of content was discussed earlier in the section on Semantics. In order to represent relational concepts linguistically, children must learn to combine words in the manner which, in their language, signals the semantic relations between words in utterances. Most children begin using two-word utterances to express relational meanings at about eighteen to twenty-four months of age.

In addition to learning the linguistic means for signaling semantic relations, children learn to use grammatical structures to modulate the basic meanings of utterances. Brown (1973) refers to these structures as *grammatic morphemes,* including forms such as plural and possessive inflections on nouns, time and person inflections on verbs, copular verbs, articles, and forms to indicate mood, aspect, and negation. Grammatical morphemes usually begin to appear when children's utterances reach a mean morpheme length of 2.0 to 2.5.

Children learn to employ various sentence forms to encode pragmatic intents as well as semantic content. Declarative and imperative structures are used to observe, comment, request, demand, insist, and so on. Negative forms express meanings such as nonexistence, rejection, and denial. Question forms are used to ask for information or confirmation of one's conclusions as well as for expressing other intents indirectly. An important aspect of language learning is acquiring skills in using the appropriate sentence forms for accomplishing one's intended purpose in speaking.

Since the late 1950s, studies of the patterns of acquisition of linguistic form have proliferated. Chomsky's theory (1957, 1965) of transformational grammar guided numerous investigations in which children's language was analyzed according to syntactic deep structures and derivational complexity of linguistic forms (Menyuk 1964, 1969; McNeill 1966a, b 1970; Bloom 1970; Leonard 1972; Morehead and Ingram 1973). During the 1970s, studies more frequently described children's utterances as semantically based, concluding that the structure of utterances is based on meaning rather than grammatical deep structure (Schlesinger 1971; Bowerman 1973a; Brown 1973). Patterns of language acquisition indicate that children learn ways to encode semantic concepts rather than ways to express grammatical concepts, such as subject and predicate of a sentence. From her analysis of the utterances of young children, Bowerman (1973a) found no justification for hypothesizing that the children in her study recognized the unity of the verb phrase in verb-direct object constructions, or that they have the abstract concept of sentence subject. She states that analysis on the basis of a generative transformational grammar model "resulted in largely gratuitous assumptions that the child had these abstract concepts" (Bowerman 1973a, p. 222). She concludes that children's utterances are described more definitively using a semantic-based model where structure is determined on the basis of the intended propositional meaning. Until children are approximately six years of age, a transformational grammar model is not needed to describe their language (Ingram 1975; de Villiers and de Villiers 1978). Bowerman (1973a) and Brown (1973) present in-depth descriptions of young children's utterances using syntax-based and semantic-based models. While details of these studies will not be included in the current discussion, readers are encouraged to be familiar with their content and conclusions.

The following discussion focuses on the relationships between meaning and linguistic form in child language. It supports the notion that children's acquisition of linguistic form is motivated and guided by their search for ways of expressing semantic concepts and pragmatic intents. Viewing the learning of linguistic structures on the basis of the meanings they convey provides a framework for remediation suggestions presented in Chapter Three.

learning to combine words

In English, semantic relations between words in utterances frequently are signaled by word order and prepositions. The effectiveness of the linear position of words in indicating relational meanings is evidenced in our ability to interpret messages conveyed through telegrams, where only high-content words are included. The recipient of a telegram reading "Conference cancelled. Meet 3:45 P.M. plane" would recognize the meaning, which in spoken communication probably would be stated as "My conference has been cancelled. Meet me on the 3:45 P.M. plane." As a further example of the influence of word order on interpretation of meaning, consider how one would interpret the phrases *big boy house* and *boy big house*. The first phrase would be expanded into *big boy's house,* and the second into *boy's big house*. The linear position of words, whether used with grammatical inflections (as in telegrams) or without inflections (as in the phrases *big boy house* and *boy big house*), signals the relational meanings of utterances.

The semantic role of nouns may be marked by prepositions. Semantic relations signaled generally by word order may be specified more exactly by a preposition. In the utterance *Put book table,* word order indicates that *table* functions as a locative. Use of a preposition such as *on, under,* or *beside* would define more specifically the nature of the locative relation. A single preposition may mark different semantic roles. The preposition *to* marks a locative relation in *He went to the store* and a beneficiary relation in *She gave the gum to Susan.* The preposition *with* marks a comitative relation in *I went with Dick* and an instrumental relation in *Joe cut it with a knife.* Table 2–4 lists prepositions commonly used to mark different semantic relations.

Combining Words: Normal Development Prior to the emergence of two-word utterances, children use single words in combination with nonlinguistic clues to signal relations among objects (including persons), actions, and conditions. As an intermediate step between one-word and multiword utterances, they often produce successive one-word utterances related to a single topic (Bloom 1973; Bloom and Lahey 1978). When reaching toward a puppy, the child may say, "Puppy. Hug." Intervening pauses, equal stress, and falling intonation patterns separate the two words. Bloom and Lahey suggest that successive one-word utterances related to a single topic indicate that the child is aware of relations among people,

TABLE 2–4
Prepositions Used to Mark Semantic Relations

SEMANTIC RELATION	PREPOSITIONS USED TO MARK THE RELATION
Locative	
Location	In, on, under, beside, behind, by, in-front-of
Direction	To, toward, from
Proximity	At, near, around, about
Instrument	With, by
Beneficiary	To, for
Comitative	With

objects, and actions or states but has not learned to express these relations linguistically. They propose that the reported variability in word order in children's early utterances (Braine 1976) may be based on descriptions of successive one-word utterances rather than descriptions of multiword utterances. When children begin using two-word utterances to express semantic relations, the order of words and prepositions mark relational concepts.

Word Order

The linear ordering of words is the first syntactic device children learn for representing linguistically the relational concepts they have formed in earlier stages of development (Bloom 1970; Schlesinger 1971; Brown 1973; Slobin 1973). Brown states:

> The child acquiring English in a huge majority of cases orders his words as they should be ordered if the semantic relations suggested by context to adults are what he intends. (Brown 1973, p. 145)

In experiments resulting in the characterization of young children's speech as "telegraphic," preservation of normal ordering of major sentence constituents is observed for both imitated and spontaneous sentences (Brown and Fraser 1964; Brown and Bellugi 1964; Brown 1973). Word order, together with contextual clues, permits listeners to interpret the intended meanings of children's telegraphic utterances. Brown (1973) explains that in two-word utterances, there are two possible orders in which words can appear; in three-word utterances, there are six. The fact that children use the word order which, in the adult version of their language, signals the intended semantic relations indicates that they are choosing to order words in a particular sequence in an effort to signal the intended meaning.

As discussed in the previous section on Semantics, the first semantic relations which children express linguistically involve actors, actions, and objects acted upon or affected by actions. These semantic roles are signaled first by word order (Brown 1973; Bowerman 1973a,b; Slobin 1973). Agentive nouns are positioned before the verb (*Mommy sit, Baby ride, Puppy bite*). Objects acted upon or affected by actions—that is, patients—appear in postverbal positions (*Ride bike, Hit ball, Kick block*). Initially, agents are animate and objects receiving or changed by the action are inanimate (Bowerman 1973b; Bloom, Miller, and Hood 1975). Not until later do nonagentive nouns appear preverbally (*Ball bounce, Car bump, Knife cut*). When action-locative relations are expressed, nouns in the locative role usually occur postverbally (*Sleep [on the] bed, Go [to the] store, Pour [it in the] cup*). When two-term utterances are combined to make three-term utterances, the linear position of noun-roles relative to the verb is maintained. Agent-action (*Baby kick*) and action-patient (*Kick ball*) become agent-action-patient (*Baby kick ball*). Agent-action (*Mommy sit*) and action-locative (*sit chair*) become agent-action-locative (*Mommy sit chair*). The preverbal position of the agent and the postverbal position of the patient or locative is maintained so that word order continues to be a linguistic device signaling the semantic relations expressed in the utterance.

Among the first state relation expressed is possessor-possession. The ordering of words is such that the possessor precedes the object possessed (*Daddy['s] chair, Baby['s] book*). When a two-term possessor-possession relation is combined with other relations, it assumes a single role in relation to the main verb in the sentence. For example, in the action-patient utterance *Drop baby('s) book*, the patient is expanded and is a two-term relation (possessor-possession):

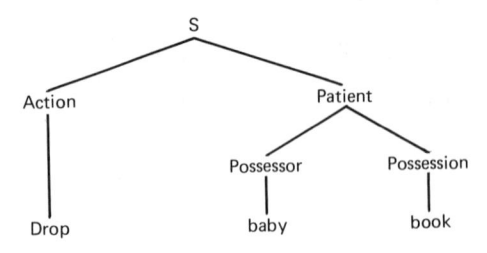

```
              S
         ╱        ╲
      Action      Patient
        │        ╱     ╲
        │   Possessor  Possession
        │       │          │
       Drop    baby       book
```

In the action-locative utterance *Sit (in) daddy('s) chair*, the locative is expanded and is a two-term relation (possessor-possession):

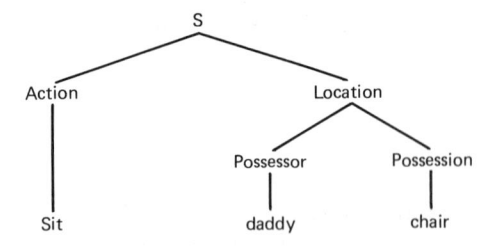

```
              S
         ╱        ╲
      Action     Location
        │        ╱     ╲
        │   Possessor  Possession
        │       │          │
       Sit    daddy       chair
```

When utterances express action events, the possessor-possession at first is likely to appear in the role of patient or locative, occurring postverbally. Since the possession usually is inanimate, it rarely serves in an agentive role in the early stages of language.

State relations expressing attribution (entity and attribute) are among the first expressed by children, although they usually do not appear until after children are expressing actions relations. When attributes appear with nouns in a nominal rather than a contrastive sense—for example, *black bear* as a label referring to a specific bear rather than a phrase contrasting a black with a white or a brown bear—the attributive word precedes the noun. The attribute-entity relation may be used to express a semantic relation with the

Chap. 2 The Foundations for Language Intervention Programs 73

main verb. In *Black doggie bite,* the agent is composed of the relation attribute-entity; in *Hit red ball,* the patient is expressed as attribute-entity. The linear position of the attribute-entity relation in action sentences will be determined by the semantic role it plays relative to the main verb. If the agent is expressed as attribute-entity, it will precede the main verb:

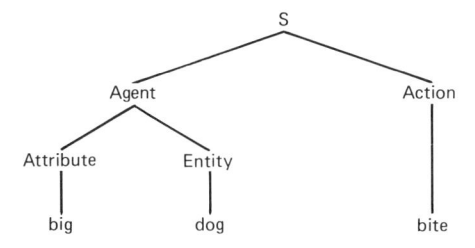

```
                    S
           ┌────────┴────────┐
         Agent             Action
       ┌───┴───┐             │
   Attribute  Entity          │
       │        │             │
      big      dog           bite
```

If the patient or locative role is expressed through the attribute-entity relation, it will appear postverbally:

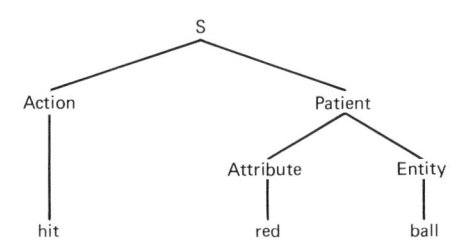

```
                    S
           ┌────────┴────────┐
         Action           Patient
           │            ┌────┴────┐
           │         Attribute  Entity
           │            │         │
          hit          red       ball
```

While English provides for attribution to be expressed in copular sentences as a predicate adjective (*The ball is red, The dog is big*), the predicate adjective construction, even with omission of the copular verb, does not appear in child language as early or as frequently as the prenominal attribute construction (Brown 1973). Therefore linear ordering in which the attribute follows the noun it describes (*Baby little, Horse brown*) appears later than ordering of the attribute before the noun (*Little baby, Brown horse*). Bloom and Lahey (1978) suggest that children use copular constructions only after they learn grammatical relations between subjects and predicates, an accomplishment achieved after the child has learned to use word order to signal semantic relations.

Entity-locative relations are expressed early in child language. Utterances referring to objects located in specific places express the entity-locative relation (*Book [is on the] table*). Statements specifying the static location of objects are less common and appear later than those referring to locative actions (Bloom, Lightbrown, and Hood 1975). Utterances referring to a change in the location of an object (*Put blocks [in the] box*) are more likely to occur than those identifying the static location of objects. When entity-locative relations appear as expressions of state, copular constructions are used, at first with omission of the copular verb (*Puppy [is on the] chair,* or *Daddy [is in the] car*). In such constructions, the locative appears after the entity whose location it specifies.

Children rarely express experiencer, instrument, beneficiary, or comitative relations until their MLU exceeds 2.0 (Brown 1973; Leonard 1976). When these relations first appear, they are likely to be signaled by word order. Nouns serving an experiencer role occur preverbally (*Mommy see,* or *I want it*). Those in an instrumental role appear postverbally (*Cut [with a] knife,* or *Draw [with a] pencil*). If the utterance contains both patient or complement and instrument relations, the instrument relation is positioned after the patient (*Cut bread [with a] knife, Draw picture [with a] pencil*). Nouns representing the beneficiary of an action or process occur postverbally (*Give [it to] mommy, Draw [it for] daddy*).

Prepositions

When children's MLU exceeds 2.0, they begin using prepositions to mark semantic relations (Brown 1973). Prepositions do not signal new relational meanings; they specify more exactly the relations encoded previously through linear positioning of words. Children learn prepositions not as a general grammatical class or as individual lexical items but according to the semantic relations that they signal.

Locative relations generally are the first marked by prepositions. Children may refer to a change in the location of the actor (*I go to school*), to a change in location of an object due to someone's actions (*Pour milk in my glass*), or to the place of an action (*He swims in the pool*). Bloom, Miller, and Hood (1975) observed that young children more frequently refer to changes in location of actors and objects than to the place of actions. Brown (1973) found *in* and *on,* used to designate specific locations in space, to be the first prepositions children use. With prepositions such as *in, on,* and *under,* they identify the place that is the goal of an action or movement. Other locative prepositions refer to directional movements rather than to a specific, observable location in space. Prepositions such as *to* (*Go to the park*), *toward* (*Walk toward the house*), and *from* (*Come from school*) are directional in nature. Some locative prepositions indicate proximity rather than directional movement or specific location. *Near* (*Stand near me*) and *at* (*He's at school*) refer to proximity of location. Children learn to mark specific locations prior to indicating general proximity. While the same prepositions are used to mark static location and locations involving actions or movements, young children make linguistic reference to action-locative relations before static locations of objects.

The prepositions *to* and *for* are learned to indicate beneficiary relations (*Give the cookie to Jack, Make a cake for daddy*). *With* is the first preposition used to mark the instrument relation (*Kick it with your foot*); subsequently, *by* is used to signal this relation (*The window was broken by a rock*). Comitative relations are marked by the preposition *with* (*Go with daddy*). Children usually do not start using prepositions to signal beneficiary, instrument, and comitative relations until after they have begun marking locative-action relations with prepositions.

In the course of normal language acquisition, children appear to learn prepositions according to the semantic relations that they signal. Stated differently, they categorize prepositions according to the semantic relations they mark. Children learning language normally may confuse prepositions within a semantic category, but they rarely show cross-category confusions (Wood 1976). They may say "I went at the park" or "He got it to the store," failing to differentiate the meanings of the locative prepositions *to* and *at*, but they are unlikely to substitute a preposition from another category for a locative preposition, so that an utterance such as *I went with the park* is rare. They may confuse the beneficiary prepositions *to* and *for*, thereby producing an utterance such as *Give this for daddy*, but cross-category errors, such as *Give this on daddy* or *Give this with daddy* are unlikely to occur. Children learn first that certain prepositions mark general semantic categories; then they learn the subcategories that indicate more subtle distinctions in meaning.

grammatical morphemes

The major meanings of utterances are represented by the semantic relations encoded in the sentence. Brown (1973) identifies a group of linguistic structures which do not change the basic meanings of utterances but modulate these meanings. He calls these linguistic forms *grammatical morphemes*. Brown states that grammatical morphemes add specificity or provide additional information to basic sentence meanings. They may orient a statement with respect to time, as is the function of alterations in verb forms, or indicate whether one or more than one instance of an object is the subject of reference, as is the function of plural markers. Brown explains that the meanings of grammatical morphemes do not exist separate from the meanings of content words and relational meanings. For example, the present progressive *-ing* form signals that an action or process identified by the verb is taking place at the time of the utterance. Past tense inflections indicate that the action or process was completed prior to the time of the utterance. Plural markers appended to nouns indicate that the item of reference exists in more than a single instance. Brown states:

It does not seem possible to think of these tunings or modulations without the things and processes they tune, whereas it does seem to be possible to conceive of the latter without the former. (1973, p. 253)

Learning to use grammatical morphemes is an important achievement in the language acquisition process, since they are an integral part of the linguistic system used by adult speakers of a language.

Grammatical Morphemes: Normal Development Once children learn to combine words to express major relational meanings, they begin adding linguistic forms which modulate the basic meanings of utterances. As their mean utterance length reaches 2.0 to 2.5 (usually between two and three years of age), children start using inflections on nouns and verbs, prepositions, copula and auxiliary verbs, and articles to add specificity and more subtle meanings to propositions they already express.

Brown (1973) describes the early acquisition of grammatical morphemes. He identifies fourteen morphemes which children learn at different rates but with substantial uniformity in their order of acquisition. Figure 2–4 shows the order of acquisition as well as the chronological ages at which three children began using these morphemes with 90 percent accuracy in contexts in which they were grammatically obligatory. Figure 2–4 also indicates the stages of development at which these fourteen morphemes were acquired. Brown's stages are defined by mean length of utterance (MLU). Mean MLU is 1.75 for Stage I; 2.25 for Stage II; 2.75 for Stage III; 3.5 for Stage IV; and 4.00 for Stage V. A study by de Villiers and de Villiers (1973) of twenty-one English-speaking children's order of acquisition of these fourteen morphemes agrees with Brown's findings. The observed order of acquisition is as follows (Brown 1973, p. 274):

1. Present progressive
2–3. *In* and *on* (learned simultaneously)
4. Plural *s*
5. Irregular past tense
6. Possessive *s*
7. Uncontractible copula
8. Articles
9. Regular past tense
10. Third person regular
11. Third person irregular
12. Uncontractible auxiliary
13. Contractible copula
14. Contractible auxiliary

Chap. 2 The Foundations for Language Intervention Programs 77

	Adam		Sarah		Eve
I (2;3)		I (2;3)		I (1;6)	
II (2;6)	Present progressive *in* *on*, plural	II (2;10)	Plural *in*, *on* Present progressive, past irregular Possessive	II (1;9)	Present progressive, *on*
III (2;11)	Uncontractible copula, past irregular	III (3;1)	Uncontractible copula Articles	III (1;11)	*in* Plural, possessive
IV (3;2)	Articles Third person irregular, possessive	IV (3;8)	Third person regular	IV (2;2)	Past regular
V (3;6)	Third person regular Past regular Uncontractible auxiliary Contractible copula Contractible auxiliary	V (4;0)	Past regular Uncontractible auxiliary Contractible copula Third person irregular Contractible auxiliary	V (2;3)	Uncontractible copula Past irregular Articles Third person regular Third person irregular Uncontractible auxiliary Contractible copula Contractible auxiliary

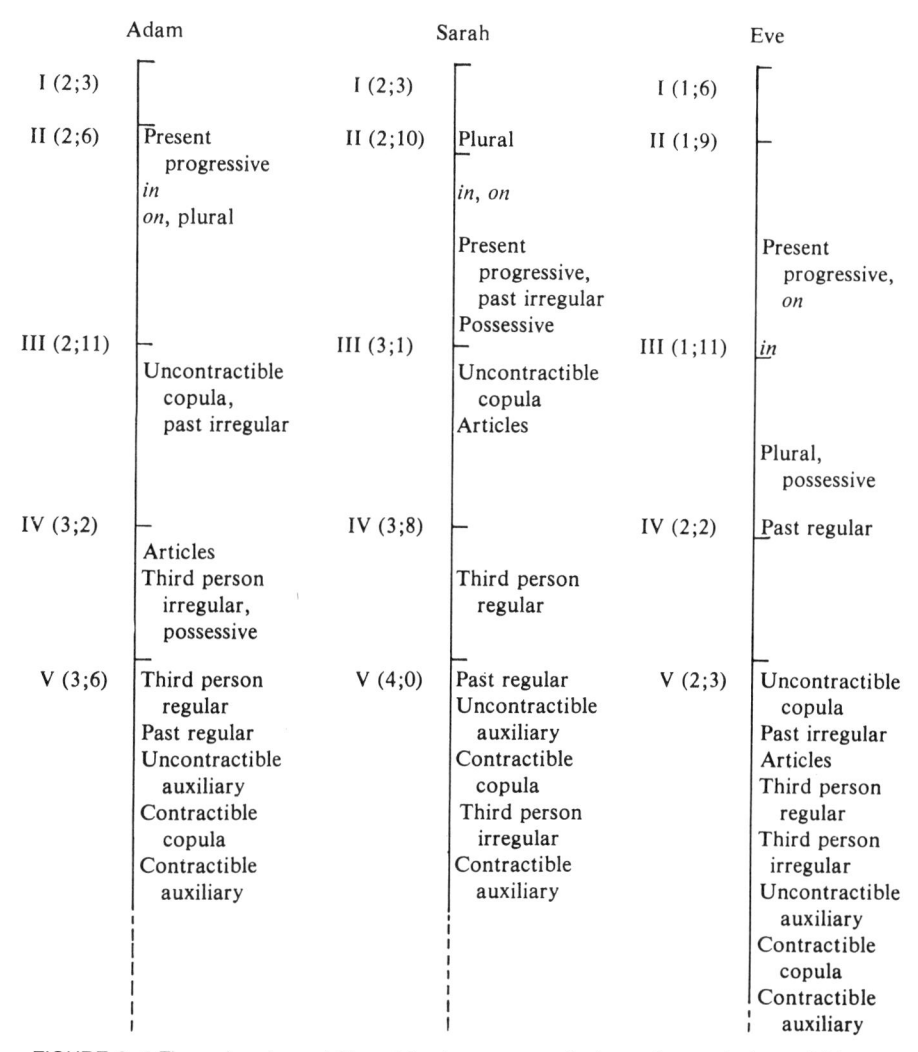

FIGURE 2-4 The order of acquisition of fourteen grammatical morphemes in three children From Brown, R. *A First Language: The Early Stages.* Cambridge, Mass.: Harvard University Press, 1973, p. 271. Reprinted by permission.

Brown (1973) identifies the fourteen morphemes first learned by most children and describes the meanings they express. Brown's discussion includes the following explanations:

>*Present Progressive:* The *-ing* form added onto verbs signals that the actions, processes, or conditions referred to by the verb are in process at the time of the utterance. The progressive form usually makes reference to actions, events, or conditions that are of temporary duration. At first, children use the *-ing* verb form without the auxiliary forms that accompany them in adult grammar (*He running* rather than *He is running*).

In and On: Children use *in* and *on* to indicate specific locations in space. *In* signals containment and is used with nouns that have internal space which can contain objects. *On* is used with nouns referring to objects that have a flat surface and are capable of supporting other objects. These two prepositions are learned together and appear to be differentiated by their containment/support contrast. *In* and *on* are used to clarify locative relations previously signaled by word order.

Plural s: The plural *s* marks the distinction between one and more than one instance of an object. In the prior stage of language development, children show an understanding that objects can occur in more than a single instance through use of words such as "more" and "another." The plural *s* often is semantically redundant, occurring with lexical items that signal more than one (*some books, those hats, more cats*).

Possessive s: The concept of possession is signaled by word order before children learn to attach the *s* to the noun representing the possessor. During earlier stages of language, children more frequently refer to alienable than to inalienable possessions. By the time they are using *s* to mark the possessor-possession relation, they make reference to inalienable as often as to alienable possessions.

Irregular and Regular Past Tense: Past tense markers signal that the event or condition of reference occurred prior to the time of the utterance. Children first use past tense in referring to events that are of very limited duration (*fell, broke, dropped*), but they soon begin to refer to past events that extend over greater spans of time (*ran, saw, played*). Irregular past tense forms generally are used before regular forms, probably because the irregular forms have higher perceptual salience. Use of simple past tense, whether expressed through irregular or regular forms, occurs several years before children express more complex past tenses such as the present perfect (*has eaten, have walked*).

Irregular and Regular Third Person: The third person regular inflection *s* signals person and number and usually is redundant with the subject of the verb to which it is attached (exceptions being nouns such as *sheep*, which do not change form to indicate plurality). The present refers to habitual activity, in contrast to the present progressive, which makes reference to events that are taking place at the time of the utterance and are of limited duration.

Uncontractible and Contractible Copula: The copula signals number, person, and tense. Number and person are also signaled by the sentence subject, making the present tense copula redundant semantically in these respects. Only when tense other than present is expressed does the copula carry nonredundant meaning. In Brown's study, the children were using past tense forms of the copula by the time they used any form with 90 percent accuracy. Therefore the copula was not totally redundant in meaning by the time its use was mastered by these children. The uncontractible copula is phonologically more simple and perceptually more salient than the contractible form. This accounts, at least in large measure, for the fact that uncontractible forms are learned earlier than contractible forms.

Articles: *The* is used to make reference to a specific instance of a class or set of objects when the speaker presupposes that the listener(s) recognizes the particular item being referred to. The article *a* is used with reference to a nonspecific or unidentified instance of a class or set of objects. Speakers are able to make the specific/nonspecific distinction effectively only if they can judge accurately what information they share with their listeners. The semantic and grammatical rules governing the use of articles in adult language are complex (see Brown 1973, pp. 340–356). In children's early use of articles, it appears that they take into account their own viewpoint but not that of a listener if it is different from their own.

Uncontractible and Contractible Auxiliary: As with the copula, auxiliary verbs add nothing to the meanings of utterances unless they signal time other than present. The uncontractible auxiliary is learned slightly earlier than the contractible form, probably for the reasons that the uncontractible copula is learned before the contractible.

Brown (1973) attempts to explain the order of acquisition of the fourteen grammatical morphemes on the basis of semantic and grammatical complexity. Both the meanings conveyed by the morphemes and their grammatical complexity influence the order in which they are learned. In addition, semantic and perceptual salience of the morpheme have an impact on order of acquisition.

learning new sentence forms

Speakers choose the type of sentence in which to couch utterances on the basis of the meaning they intend to convey and the context in which they are speaking. The sentence form assists listeners in recognizing the purpose for which the speaker is speaking and often reflects important information about the social context and the relationship between speaker and listener. Certain sentence types permit speakers to encode more complex semantic notions. Through processes of conjoining and embedding, speakers can signal relational meanings that are not represented in a single simple sentence. Learning to use a variety of sentence types is an important linguistic achievement.

New Sentence Forms: Normal Development The majority of children's early utterances are simple, declarative forms. When their mean utterance length approaches 3.0 morphemes (usually around age three), they begin using negations, yes/no questions, wh-questions, and imperatives, and they learn to perform the linguistic operations neccessary for formulating these utterance types. With an expansion in the sentence forms they can generate, children are more effective in specifying their intents and in altering the form of their utterances to fit the situation. Subsequently they learn to coordinate sentence constituents and propositions and to embed one sentence within another to formulate complex sentences.

Negation

Children's earliest statements usually are affirmative, referring to things that actually exist and to events that actually occur. Their earliest expressions of negation encode the semantic notions of nonexistence, or disappearance, rejection, and denial, followed soon by expressions of cessation and prohibition. Initially, a single word, most often *no,* is used to express negation. When children begin using two-word utterances, they encode negation syntactically. In early multiword utterances, negation is expressed through combining *no* with a content word. For example, *no book* may signal the disappearance of a child's book. *No run* may express that someone has ceased running. *No juice* may encode rejection of juice being offered to the child. *No talk* may be a statement of prohibition in which the child forbids someone to talk.

Bloom, Miller, and Hood (1975) observed that children's early negative sentences usually were composed of a negative marker (most often *no*) and an object noun or verb. To reduce utterance complexity, children at first omitted the subject or agentive noun in negative utterances. When they increased utterance complexity to include the sentence subject and a negative marker plus the verb, the negative marker usually appeared between the subject and the verb. Sentences such as *Baby no drink* and *Mommy no talk* appeared.

Bellugi (1967) found that fairly early in language learning, children begin using forms in addition to *no* to mark negation. Early-appearing forms included *not, can't,* and *don't.* Initially, *can't* and *don't* appeared as lexical items indicating negation. Not until mean utterance length reached approximately 3.4 were *can't* and *don't* used as negative auxiliary forms.

Imperatives

Imperative sentences, used to request, demand, or suggest an action response from the addressee, usually appear in English as utterances in which the implied subject, *you,* is not expressed. Children's early communicative acts serving an instrumental or regulatory function are intended to accomplish purposes similar to those which older children and adults express through imperative sentence forms. In the initial stages of sentence construction, children produce many subjectless sentences in issuing requests or demands. While these utterances appear in the same form as adult imperative sentences, one cannot attribute to young children the linguistic knowledge which underlies the adult's production of imperative constructions. Brown (1973) points out that young children at first produce declarative and interrogative as well as imperative sentences without expressed subjects. Only when they use subjectless sentences exclusively in an imperative sense should they be given credit for knowing imperative syntax.

Imperative constructions are frequent in children's speech throughout the preschool years. Garvey (1975) found that until about four and one-half years of age, children's requests for actions usually are expressed in imperative forms. Between the ages of four and one-half and five and one-half years, children begin presenting more of their requests indirectly, using interrogative and declarative constructions, such as *Will you shut the door* or *I like chocolate candy* in place of *Shut the door* or *Give me some chocolate candy.* However, even at this older age level, direct requests stated in imperative constructions occur more frequently than indirect requests couched in other sentence forms. Children are likely to use politeness markers such as *please* (*Please open the window*) before they change the form of sentences to make a request indirectly (*Can you open the window?*). Garvey suggests that the form of children's requests "reflects an intersection of social and linguistic competence" (1975, p. 62).

Question Forms

Question forms are used to confirm or refute one's observations and conclusions, and to seek unknown information. Children begin giving discriminating responses to yes/no and wh-questions before these question forms emerge in their speech (Brown 1968; Horgan 1977; Rodgon 1979). Rodgon (1979) found that children between one and one-half and two years of age discriminate between yes/no and wh-questions directed to them. The children in her study answered *yes* or *no* to questions whose form called for a yes/no response but not to questions seeking a missing constituent, that is, wh-questions. Rodgon concluded that these children recognized which question forms called for a yes/no response and which asked for other information.

Children's early utterances seeking confirmation or denial of their conclusions are likely to be declarative forms spoken with rising intonation. *This is a cup?* or *Baby is sleeping?* may be used to ask the listener to agree or disagree with the proposition. Until mean utterance length approaches 3.0, children do not begin transposing sentence constituents (*Is baby sleeping?*) to transform declarative into interrogative sentence forms to ask yes/no questions (Brown 1973). Tag questions (*Baby is sleeping, isn't she?* or *Daddy isn't gone, is he?*), formulated through more complex derivational processes, are not used until children are at least four years old (Brown and Hanlon 1970).

In English, wh-questions serve as requests for unknown grammatical constituents or semantic relations. The wh-word stands for the unknown constituent; together with the verb, it specifies what information is being sought. After children are encoding certain semantic relations in declarative sentence forms, they begin to respond appropriately to wh-questions in which the missing constituent plays one of the semantic roles they know how to express in declarative utterances (Rodgon 1979).

Brown (1968, 1973) describes the development of wh-question forms in child language. *What's that?* or *What dat?* is the only wh-question which appears frequently prior to the time that children have MLU's of 2.75 to 3.0. Brown indicates that this early question form seems to be an independent routine, produced as an unanalyzed phrase. He observed a pattern in the development of syntactic patterns used in constructing wh-questions. In adult forms, the wh-word representing the missing constituent is preposed so that it appears as the first word in the sentence; additionally, the sentence subject and the auxiliary verb are transposed. Brown found that children learn to prepose the wh-word before they transpose the subject and auxiliary, so that as an intermediate step on the way to adult interrogative forms, they produce questions such as *What his name is?* and *Why you can't open it?* Subsequently they learn to transpose constituents appropriately and formulate wh-questions correctly (*What is his name? Why can't you open it?*).

The order of acquisition of wh-questions is influenced by meaning. Ervin-Tripp (1970) found that children respond correctly to *who, what,* and *where* questions much earlier than to *when, why,* and *how* questions. This order of acquisition cannot be attributed to differences in grammatical complexity, since *when, why* and *how* questions are no more grammatically complex than *who, what,* and *where* questions. Children learn *who, what,* and *where* earlier because they make reference to people, objects, actions, and locations, which are concepts children formulate before they learn about time, cause, and manner.

Complex Sentences

As MLU reaches 3.0, generally at about three years of age, children begin expressing more than one proposition within a single sentence. To accomplish this, they produce complex sentences, which Limber describes as "any sentence with more than one verb" (1973, p. 171). Through the syntactic processes of coordination and embedding, they program two or more simple sentences, that is, separate propositions, into one sentence.

COORDINATION. Coordination of two simple sentences can be accomplished in several ways. The conjunctive *and* is first used to conjoin simple sentences (*I like cake and John likes cake* or *That dog barks and that dog bites*). Subsequently, simple sentences are coordinated using the disjunctive *or* (*I will sing or you will sing*), a causal form such as *because* (*I hit him because he broke my car*); forms such as *and then* to indicate temporal succession (*I went inside and then he closed the door*); contrastive terms such as *but* (*I called him but he didn't answer*); and conditional forms such as *if . . . then* (*If you read to me then I'll read to you*). There is semantic continuity between the simple sentences that are coordinated. Bloom and Lahey (1978) explain that sentences to be coordinated refer to conditions or events that are related in time and/or space. Each of the sentences has meaning separate from the other, and neither is changed in meaning when they are conjoined.

Children learn to eliminate the redundancy in two simple sentences to be coordinated, thereby producing utterances in which constituents are coordinated. When two sentences have an identical element serving in the same semantic or syntactic role, this element can be deleted in one sentence and the nonidentical parts of the sentence can be linked with *and*. Through this process, the sentences *Tom jumped* and *Tom ran* become *Tom jumped and ran*. Similarly, *Joe sang* and *Mary sang* become *Joe and Mary sang*. Constituents to be coordinated from two simple sentences must be structurally identical but lexically distinct (Brown 1973). Brown points out that in order to construct coordinations with deletions, children must have knowledge of sentence constituents, constituent types, and semantic or syntactic roles. They must be able to identify sentence elements which are identical and those which are nonidentical but structurally matched.

Whether coordination of full sentences (*John came home and John played*) is learned before coordination of constituents with redundant elements deleted from one sentence (*John came home and played*) is an unsettled issue. The de Villiers (1978) cite studies of coordination in spontaneous utterances and in elicited imitations indicating that children begin conjoining simple sentences using *and* before they start to use reduced coordinations. They also point out that in some studies of spontaneous speech, coordination with deletion has been observed in children's speech several months before full sentences are conjoined. Additional research will be necessary to decide this question.

EMBEDDING. In addition to coordination, children use embedding to express more than one proposition in a single sentence. Brown (1973) explains that embedding is a syntactic process by which one sentence becomes a grammatical constituent of another or one proposition plays a certain semantic role in another proposition. Children's first embedded constructions have propositions serving as object complements. Utterances such as *I want (to) go outside, I don't like (to) sit by you, Watch me jump,* and *Look at the puppy run* are the types of utterances that reflect embedding in children's early language. Limber (1973) points out that in children's speech, object complements appear as unmarked infinitives (*See me break this*), marked infinitives (*I like to play*), wh-clauses (*I know where daddy is*), or full sentences (*I know you have my ball*). Rarely do young children use *-ing* complement forms such as *I like playing ball.*

After children learn to use embedding to formulate object complements, they begin using relative clauses. Propositions stated in relative clauses do not function as major grammatical or semantic constituents in relation to the main verb of the sentence. They add additional information about a major sentence constituent. Brown (1973) states that relative clauses generally function as attributes, providing more definitive information about a noun which serves as a major sentence constituent. For example, in the sentence *I like the shirt you gave me,* the relative clause *you gave me* identifies the particular shirt referred to. Limber (1973) states that adverbial relative clauses (*I'll do it when we get home* or *You do it like I do it*) are among the first types of relative clause constructions that children use. Brown (1973) and Limber (1973) note that children do not use subject complements (*Playing cards is fun* or *To sing is fun*) and relative clauses attached to subject nouns (*The boy who hit me ran away* or *The girl from Dallas was not here*) until considerably later than they use object complements or relative clauses attached to object nouns.

syntax: examples of disordered development

To report that the verbal output of many language-disordered children is characterized by deficiencies in linguistic form is no revelation to persons who have dealt with these children. Acceptance of the theory of transformational grammar led to numerous studies comparing normal and language-deviant children on the basis of the linguistic structure of their utterances, and to the development of assessment procedures that distinguish language disordered from normal-speaking children.

Using a transformational grammar model for analyzing spontaneous utterances, Menyuk (1964, 1969), Leonard (1972), and Morehead and Ingram (1973) found that preschool children with deviant language could be distinguished from those with normal language on the basis of their use of linguistic forms. Menyuk concluded that the most significant factor separating the two groups of children was the "ability to determine complete sets of rules that are used to generate and differentiate structures at any level of grammar" (1964, p. 119). Leonard found that language-deviant children differed from their normal peers primarily in frequency of usage of syntactic and morphological structures. The two groups did not differ in the number of deviant forms used or in the developmental level of structures used correctly. Morehead and Ingram found that normal and deviant-speaking preschool children differed in number of major syntactic categories per construction type and in onset and acquisition time for base syntax, transformation, construction types, and minor lexical categories such as pronouns, prepositions, modals, and demonstratives. They concluded that the primary differences in the two groups were the rate of acquisition and the creativity in using linguistic forms. In a study comparing the acquisition of grammatical morphemes by normal and language-disordered children, Johnston and Schery (1976) found that the two groups "learned the same forms, in much the same order, and with the same general relationships to overall language development level as indexed by sentence length" (pp. 256–57). Compared with normal speakers, the children with deviant language progressed more slowly from initial use to complete mastery of grammatical morphemes.

Most studies based on a transformational grammar model treat the learning of language forms as the learning of rules of grammar. The relationship between meaning and form is not a prominent factor in describing the children's patterns of learning linguistic structures. Inconsistent use of linguistic structures by language-disordered children is noted, but the relationship between the correct or incorrect appearance of a structure and meaning is not emphasized.

A few studies have considered the relationship between meaning and form. Menyuk (1969) observed that while language-deviant children frequently omit sentence constituents that are grammatically obligatory, the meaning of the sentence usually is interpretable because the omitted constituents are semantically redundant. Cole (1976) found that preschool children with language disorders differed from normal speakers in frequency of omissions of sentence constituents whose meaning was apparent from the context but not in omission of constituents whose absence made the meaning uninterpretable. In a study of the use of certain grammatical morphemes by preschool children with language disorders, Wood (1976) found inconsistencies in correct and incorrect usage. She found that semantic and perceptual salience and grammatic and semantic complexity appeared to influence the language-disordered children's use of grammatical morphemes. Some of the language-disordered children continued to rely on word order to mark semantic relations rather than on use of grammatically obligatory morphemes to signal such relations. Their errors appeard to be not in the ability to express relational notions but in learning the grammatical morphemes which signal their meaning.

Earlier in this chapter, examples were given of evidences of disordered development in language use and in language content. Deficits in communication such as those described may be compounded by deficiencies in learning of linguistic form. Language-disordered children evidence deficits in linguistic form when they fail to learn structures which encode pragmatic intents and semantic notions that they communicate nonlinguistically or through combining words and phrases with contextual clues.

summary of syntax

Children must learn to use linguistic structures to convey their intentions and to represent concepts if they are to use language normally. Word order is the first syntactic device learned to signal relational notions. Children then learn to use grammatical morphemes to mark relational concepts and to modulate the basic meaning of utterances. They learn to alter sentence forms and to select the sentence type that best encodes the message they wish to transmit. The sequence and patterns of learning of linguistic form appears to be influenced by the meanings which various structures signal and by the semantic and grammatical complexity of the forms.

Numerous studies have shown significant differences in normally developing and language-deviant children in terms of linguistic forms used. In order to address the needs of many children with language disorders, intervention programs must include plans and strategies for teaching language form. In Chapter Three, suggestions are given for integrating the teaching of language form with improving language use. Additionally, readers will be referred to sources that describe intervention strategies for teaching language form.

○ LANGUAGE ASSESSMENT

Assessment is an important part of language intervention programs. The purposes of language assessment include identifying children who are not learning language normally and describing their language proficiencies and deficiencies so that appropriate intervention plans can be designed. Screening procedures should locate children whose language is deficient so that they can be seen for more thorough study. The product of the more in-depth assessment should be a description of the child's language in terms of use, content, and form. The description should not be limited to a report of a child's vocabulary, utterance length, sentence types, or other aspects of language in terms of age norms. Such data may be of assistance in recognizing the existence of certain language deficits, but knowing that a child's vocabulary is at a 2 year, 6 months level on a particular test or that mean utterance length is 3.4 morphemes provides little direction for remediation planning. A description should tell what the child knows about language and what she or he does with language when called upon to use it under different circumstances. No firm line of demarcation can be drawn between the point at which assessment ends and intervention begins. Throughout the remediation process, clinicians should continue to note pertinent information about the child's language behavior and adapt intervention procedures according to their revised understandings of the child's facility with language.

A detailed presentation on language assessment is beyond the purview of this book. Other sources should be consulted for a comprehensive treatment of assessment. Snyder (1981) considers bases and tools for assessing prelinguistic communicative development. Scott (1978) discusses important considerations in evaluating the development of infants. Uzgiris and Hunt (1975) provide developmental scales and suggest procedures for assessing infant development. Siegel and Broen (1976) address the dimensions of language to be included in an in-depth evaluation, and discuss the usefulness of standardized and nonstandardized procedures. Miller (1978) presents an excellent discussion of the development of a comprehensive assessment plan, evaluation procedures, and interpretation of language data gathered during the assessment process. Bloom and Lahey (1978) discuss a broad range of factors that should be considered in selecting processes and tools to be used in efforts to describe children's language for the purpose of planning intervention. Miller (1981) provides plans and procedures for assessing children's language production. Schery (1981) discusses important considerations for selecting assessment strategies. The following discussion addresses in a cursory manner some considerations the author believes are important in assessing child language. The discussion reflects the author's contention that a clinician needs to know how a child uses language in realistic communication situations in order to describe the child's language proficiencies and deficiencies for the purposes of setting appropriate goals and selecting effective strategies for intervention.

the assessment process

The clinician's responsibility in assessing language is to come up with a comprehensive description of the child's typical patterns of language, and to identify factors which facilitate or inhibit the child's learning and use of language. The principal sources of information about a child's abilities and disabilities are (1) reports from parents or others who spend substantial amounts of time with the child, (2) the clinician's direct observations of the child using language under a variety of circumstances, and (3) results of standardized tests. For children who have experienced medical problems or have received assistance from other professionals, reports should be obtained from physicians, physical therapists, occupational therapists, psychologists, teachers, social workers, and others who have been involved with the child. All children with deviant language should have an audiological assessment so that information about the functioning of the auditory system can be included in the description of the child's communicative functioning, and considered when intervention strategies are selected. The person responsible for assessment should gather and integrate the information available from all sources to formulate a comprehensive picture of the child's language skills. The key to effective assessment is a clinician who has a thorough understanding of normal language learning, is a keen observer, knows how to elicit pertinent information and behavior from parents and children, and is able to analyze data and integrate information so that patterns of language learning and use are evident.

Information from Parents Clinicians can gain valuable insights into a child's language if they are skilled in listening to, questioning, and analyzing what parents (or other familiar adults) say. Parents should recognize that their contributions are a valuable part of the assessment process so that they will provide as complete information about their child as possible. Clinicians should be familiar with techniques for interviewing, such as those provided by McDonald (1962) and Edinburg, Zinberg, and Kelman (1975).

Parents generally come to the professional with concerns about their child's current condition or behavior. Initially, they may talk more freely about their immediate concerns than about past conditions or problems. By listening to parents' reports, the clinician often gains clues about the level of development at which the child functions, and about the nature and extent of the language deficit. After listening to the parents' descriptions of the problem, the clinician can follow with questions relative to the use, content, and structure of the child's language. Examples of the types of questions that elicit information about the uses to which a child puts language include the following:

> How does Tommy let you know what he wants?
>
> What does he do when he wants you to do something? (to move out of his way? to sit down? to open a jar? to draw a picture?)
>
> What does he do to get you to play favorite games with him? How does he go about engaging you in such activities?
>
> What does Tommy do when he wants you to pay attention to him or to look at something of interest to him?
>
> What are his ways of letting you know how he feels about something that is going on? How does he signal to you that he is happy? (sad? angry? excited? frightened? tired?)
>
> When playing alone, does he make noises as though he is entertaining himself or talking to himself?
>
> During play, does he say things or make sounds that are associated with whatever he is doing? (motor noises? animal sounds? conversation-like talk?)
>
> What kinds of descriptive comments does Tommy make, either to himself or to you, about objects or events?
>
> Does he report to you on things he has done, has seen done, or wants to do outside of the immediate setting?
>
> Does he ask you for information? (names of items or people? labels or explanations of events or actions? locations of objects?)

Questions such as the following may bring out useful information about the child's conversational skills:

> When you say something to Tommy, how does he acknowledge that you have spoken to him?
>
> When he addresses you, does he usually say or do something to indicate that he is speaking to you or to get your attention before he says what he has to say?
>
> When addressing someone or carrying on a conversation, does Tommy take turns speaking, or is he likely to begin talking while someone else is speaking?

Chap. 2 The Foundations for Language Intervention Programs   89

> When he says something to you, does he usually expect you to respond or at least to acknowledge that you have heard him? What does he do if you don't respond?
>
> When you say something to which he gives a response, does his response usually match or correspond to what you said to him?
>
> If he doesn't understand or hasn't heard you, does he ask for clarification?
>
> If you don't answer him correctly or if you question what he has said, does he try to clarify what he has said? If so, how? (repeat what he has said? reword his utterance? add new information?)
>
> When he asks or tells you something, does he usually give you enough information so that you understand what he means?
>
> When asking or telling you something, is what he says well enough organized so that you can follow his train of thought?
>
> Does he use more polite forms in talking to adults or to strangers than when talking to his peers or siblings? Does he seem to realize that he can phrase things in certain ways when talking to his friends or siblings but needs to phrase them differently when talking to adults?

In conjunction with or in addition to questions such as those in the preceding lists, the clinician may seek information about the content and structure of a child's language in day-to-day situations. Such information may have been revealed by the parents' examples of what the child would be likely to say under various circumstances. More specific inquiries about the content and structure of language might include questions such as the following:

> Does Tommy know the names for most familiar objects and people? If not, how does he make you know about whom or what he is talking?
>
> Does he use words to talk about actions, such as what he or someone else is doing?
>
> What kinds of things does he tell about objects, people, or events? (attributes? locations? time? causation? functions?)
>
> Is it usually necessary for you to see or know what he is talking about in order to understand what he means?
>
> Does he put several words together to ask for something he wants? (to tell about things he is doing? to tell you what to do?)
>
> How long are his typical sentences?
>
> Does he leave words out of sentences?
>
> Does he use complex sentences, or are his sentences usually simple?
>
> Does he use pronouns correctly in referring to people and things?
>
> Does he use words or grammatical forms that refer to time? (words such as *later, yesterday, tomorrow,* as well as past or future verb tenses?)
>
> Does he use several sentences in making explanations?

It is best to state questions in an open-ended manner so that parents give descriptions and examples of their child's language rather than yes-no responses to the questions. If the parents' responses do not include examples of the child's language, the clinician should ask for them. Information relative to several aspects of the child's language may be revealed in examples, thus eliminating the need to ask some other questions. For example, if parents have said that their child would say something like "Me like cookie," "Her broke cup," and "Him silly," there would be no need to ask if the child uses pronouns correctly or leaves words out of sentences, since this information is evident from the examples the parent has given. The clinician's knowledge of normal developmental patterns will serve as a guide in selecting questions. If the parent has already reported that the child has just begun using a few single words, few if any questions would be asked about sentence length and complexity and about conversational skills.

Some clinicians prefer to talk in detail to parents before seeing the child, while others choose to observe the child before talking to the parents. The order of events will vary according to the clinician's prior information about the child, the availability of the parent or other familiar adult, the preferences and needs of parents, and the clinician's preferences. The author generally elects to talk to parents briefly to obtain a general statement of their concerns, then to observe the child, and then to seek additional information from the parent based on the observations of the child. Talking with parents before seeing the child provides clues to the nature of the problem and therefore guides the initial observations; it also gives parents opportunities to express their concern and may make them realize that they are contributing to the assessment process. From observing the child, certain questions may be answered and others raised so that the subsequent interviews of the parents are more directed. The author generally finds it useful to have the parents participate in the initial session, or to report to the parents the nature of the child's language behavior and to ask if this behavior corresponds with what they see in living with the child on a daily basis.

Certain information about the child's history should be obtained to assist the clinician in identifying important patterns of development and possible causes of problems. Bangs (1968) and Berry (1969) provide examples of forms to guide clinicians in obtaining and recording pertinent background information. Knowledge of the family history, prenatal conditions, birth history, past and present medical conditions, verbal and nonverbal developmental patterns, and social-emotional development may assist the clinician in understanding the child's present condition. *Intervention Strategies for High Risk Infants and Children,* edited by Tjossem (1976), provides useful information about conditions that are likely to lead to developmental disabilities, including language disorders.

If adults other than parents spend substantial amounts of time with a child, they generally can provide pertinent information about communication skills. With the permission of the parents or guardian, clinicians should seek from others familiar with the child information similar to that asked of parents about the child's behavior. The clinician may ask for written reports or may interview the individual, either in person or by telephone. The author has found that teachers or child-care workers usually provide more complete information in a conversation than when they are asked to provide a written statement. In a conversation with the teacher or other adult, the clinician has an opportunity to ask clarifying questions about information given and to seek examples which may reveal important patterns of language behavior. Just as with parents, other adults are more likely to try to give comprehensive information if they realize that their contributions will assist in identifying the child's needs and in providing the types of intervention that will be most helpful to the child. The clinician should explain why the information is being sought and to what use it will be put.

The Observation Process Observations of the child using language usually serve as the primary source of information necessary for making judgments about the child's language abilities and disabilities. The clinician will have only limited exposure to the child's language behavior and must make decisions on the basis of analyses of this sample of language. The clinician should strive to collect samples of language behavior which reveal typical patterns of language content, form, and use.

The context and procedures used in gathering the sample influence the child's language behavior. Language elicited in highly structured contexts, such as in formal testing, often is not typical of the language a child uses in low-structure situations (Dever 1972; Prutting, Gallagher, and Mulac 1975). Longhurst and Grubb (1974) found that utterances elicited in tightly structured tasks are shorter and less complex than those children use in more loosely structured contexts. Miller (1978) states, "... the more structured the elicitation session, the less varied the resultant language in terms of the variety of structures and meanings expressed" (p. 293). Fey, Leonard, and Wilcox (1980) found that utterances of language-disordered preschool children vary in some dimensions according to the age of the listener. Findings such as these point out the importance of considering situational influences in setting up language assessments. This author's preference is to obtain samples of language behavior in a free-speech context, attempting to create or allow situations that approximate as closely as possible those in which the child is likely to use language in the everyday world. Miller (1981) suggests useful procedures for creating a context in which to collect free-speech samples of children's language. Lee (1974) discusses ways to elicit speech samples that are likely to include a variety of utterance structures.

Clinicians should see children in situations that are natural and interesting or important to the child. When possible, they should observe a child in the day-care setting, school, or home; in both familiar and novel activities with peers and adults; in natural interactions with family members; in solitary play; and in encounters with unfamiliar people, objects, and events. It often is not possible for the clinician to be with a child in multiple locations. Assessments usually are done in a clinical setting, removed from the child's normal environment. It is the clinician's challenge to organize the situation so that it is as natural as possible for the child.

Observing the child's interactions with familiar people may elicit usual language behavior more readily than if the child is taken into a new situation with an unfamiliar adult. Attention to the child's interactions with family members in the waiting room may provide useful information about language. Parents or siblings may be brought into the room to do things with the child that he or she is likely to enjoy and take part in. Since older persons usually adapt their behavior to meet the child's needs, clinicians can gain insights into the child's communication skills by observing the way that familiar adults or older siblings adjust when dealing with the child. Varying degrees of instruction may be necessary to guide the nature of family members' interactions with the child in the assessment setting. Knowing that language is the focus of attention in that situation, parents may quiz the child in an effort to elicit speech. They are likely to ask the child to name items, give colors, count, or perform other specific verbal tasks. If such quizzing dominates the interaction, the clinician may tell parents something like "I want to see how Jane communicates with you under normal circumstances. Just play with her as you would at home. Don't do anything special to try to make her talk." With siblings, it may be important for the clinician to be especially unobtrusive in observing so that the interactions will be as natural as possible rather than contrived performances for the clinician. If the initial interactions do not create communication episodes which the clinician feels are important to observe, parents or siblings may be asked to set up specific circumstances that call for particular types of language behavior from the child. For example, they may point out an item the child likes but cannot reach so that the child needs to ask for it; do something that will cause the child to protest; ignore the child so that he or she needs to perform some act to call for their attention; or fail to understand so that the child needs to clarify his or her intent. The point of having the child interact with a familiar person is to provide the clinician with samples of how the child uses language in such interactions.

The clinician may find that an adequate range of language behaviors are elicited or demanded of the child in the joint activities with parents or siblings. If this does not occur, or if parents or other children are not available to take part in the session, the clinician must participate directly in order to create situations that reveal the desired information about various aspects of the child's language. Even if the child-family interactions provide a broad sample of the child's language behavior, the clinician, as an unfamiliar adult, may intercede to see if the child's language is different with unfamiliar and familiar persons. The extent to which the clinician acts as an observer or a participant will depend on what information is being sought, whether the desired language behaviors are being elicited or demanded, and the availability of familiar adults or children to take part in the assessment process.

It is important to determine how a child uses language for purposes other than interpersonal interactions. The clinician should find out if and how the child employs language for organizing what is going on, directing his or her own behavior, creating make-believe situations, and representing events and conditions. This may be accomplished by observing the child playing alone. Also, parallel play situations where the parents, siblings, or clinician engage themselves in activities of interest to the child may be set up. Persons playing alongside the child may comment on what they are doing, have just done, or are about to do; assume the role and talk for various dolls with which they are playing; comment on some attribute or condition of a toy; verbalize a feeling or attitude toward what is happening; or otherwise comment on their activities or on events around them. Such verbalizations should not dominate the situation and should not be used to engage the child in interactions. However, another person's behaving in this manner may set the stage for the child to use vocalizations and verbalizations as a part of his or her activities.

The nature of the assessment situation described in the preceding paragraphs contrasts significantly with highly structured conditions in which the clinician administers standardized tests and the child is restricted to performing specific tasks in the manner prescribed by the test. Noting how the child behaves during structured testing may reveal some useful information about the ability to use language in some contexts, but it reveals very little about the function, content, and form of the child's language in the various circumstances in which language is needed and employed in daily living. Especially for young children, the nature of interactions and the communicative demands imposed during test administrations are likely to be far removed from the interactions and demands for language in natural settings. The clinician is more likely to get samples of the child's usual language behavior if the circumstances for language use in the assessment process are natural for the child than if the situation is stilted and the child is forced to take part in highly structured, clinician-dominated tasks.

Recording Speech Samples Making an accurate recording of the child's utterances and of the contexts in which they occur is an important part of the language assessment process. Miller (1981) gives suggestions for making audiotape, videotape, and written recordings of language, and for transcribing tapes of children's language. Regardless of the method of recording used, the transcript of the sample of language to be analyzed must include not only precisely what the child says but also information about the linguistic and nonlinguistic context surrounding utterances. The linguistic context includes utterances, whether produced by the child or by someone else, that precede and follow a given utterance. The nonlinguistic context includes objects and people associated with the utterance; gestures or actions of the child or someone else; visual pursuits related to the utterance; facial expressions; and auditory stimuli to which the utterance is related. Unless utterances are considered within their context, their propositional and referential meanings may be misconstrued, their intended effect on the listener may be unclear, and the appropriateness of their content and form may not be evident.

Analyzing Speech Samples The nature of the analysis of free-speech samples will be determined by the information that the analyzer is seeking. Numerous guidelines and procedures for analysis of language use, meaning, and form have been proposed. Some result in assigning a developmental age score, a percentile rank, or a standard score to a given aspect of language. These are *norm-referenced* descriptions, which compare a child with other children. Norm-referenced procedures are more useful for identifying children who may need intervention than for determining remediation goals and strategies for a particular child. Some systems for analyzing free-speech samples result in *criterion-referenced* descriptions. They compare a child's performance to an identified standard of performance for a particular aspect of behavior and indicate how well-established that behavior is for the child. Criterion-referenced procedures provide information useful for developing goals for intervention because they assist in identifying the developmental stage at which a child is functioning in a particular aspect of behavior, and thereby guide the clinician toward setting goals that reflect subsequent stages in the developmental sequence. Gorth and Hambleton (1972), Bloom and Lahey (1978), Scott (1978), Prutting (1979), and Miller (1981) discuss the use of criterion-referenced descriptions in assessment and intervention planning.

Several systems for analyzing the communicative functions or illocutionary force of children's spontaneous utterances have been devised. Greenfield and Smith (1976) identify functional categories that can describe children's early communicative vocalizations. Halliday (1977) provides a system that he found useful for coding the functions of his son's early communicative acts. Dore (1975) proposes categories of speech acts that can be used to describe children's one-word utterances. Dore (1977, 1978) presents speech act categories that identify the illocutionary force of children's utterances. Dale (1980) provides a coding system for the functions of children's utterances. While these systems for describing the communicative functions of children's utterances have been used primarily with children learning language normally, they can be applied in analyzing the communicative behavior of children with deficient language.

Procedures for describing children's conversational skills are available, primarily in literature investigating normal language learning. Moerk (1975) suggests categories that describe mother-child interactions involving preschool children. Prutting and others (1978) provide a system for coding children's communicative acts, responses to prior requests, and discourse topics during adult-child discourse. Rodgon, Jankowski, and Alenskas (1977) give categories for coding dyadic interactions between parent and child. Blank and Franklin (1980) provide a system for assessing dialogic behavior of preschoolers. Dale (1980) suggests a system for coding the dialogue status of utterances. Garvey (1975) shows how requests and acknowledgments of requests can be categorized as they appear in conversational episodes. Gallagher (1981) describes a means of coding contingent queries that are unsolicited. Garvey (1977) has a system for analyzing requests for clarification during conversation. Musselwhite, St. Louis, and Penick (1980) suggest ways to code certain types of communicative interactional attempts among school-age children, and their system could be adapted for use with younger children. Chapman's (1981) review of procedures for investigating children's language use identifies many systems for analyzing this aspect of language and discusses their application in the assessment of child language.

Free-speech samples can be analyzed to describe the referential and propositional meanings of utterances. One measure of children's knowledge of referential meanings of words is the type-token ratio (TTR), which shows the relationship between the number of different types of words used and the total number of words in a language sample. Templin (1957) designed a procedure for calculating the TTR in a 50-utterance sample. The TTR serves as one measure of vocabulary diversity. Bloom and Lahey (1978) suggest ways to identify content categories represented in children's utterances. Single words are separated into nouns and relational words. Relational words are then placed in content categories, such as existence, recurrence, attribution, possession, action, locative-action, and so on. Bloom and Lahey state that the type of analysis they propose assists in determining whether children need to learn to use words in a wider range of contexts. Miller (1981) proposes a semantic field analysis as a means of recognizing the meaning categories represented by the words children use in free-speech samples. Miller states, "... semantic field analysis gives us another way of talking about the diversity and complexity of the child's vocabulary in terms of both number of meaning categories and different words within categories" (1981, p. 42).

To describe the propositional or relational meanings of utterances, children's utterances can be analyzed to determine which semantic relations they encode in free-speech samples. Brown's (1973) sets of semantic relations that are prevalent in early two- and three-word utterances provide a system for describing relational meanings encoded by those at early stages of language development. MacDonald and Blott (1974) show how children's utterances can be analyzed according to semantic relations and how the results can serve as a basis for planning remediation. Leonard, Bolders, and Miller (1976) present a modification of Fillmore's (1968) case grammar categories for use in coding the semantic relations encoded by preschool children. Clancy, Jacobsen, and Silva (1976) devised a system for describing semantic relations expressed in conjoined sentences and present data related to the sequence of development of semantic relations in more complex utterances. Miller (1981) discusses the application of systems of analysis proposed by Brown and by Clancy, Jacobsen, and Silva for assessment and remediation planning.

Numerous systems have been developed for analyzing the linguistic form of samples of children's language. Brown's (1973) procedures for deriving mean length of utterance (MLU) frequently are employed. Miller (1981) presents a slight variation of Brown's procedures and discusses the significance of MLU in language assessments. Lee (1974) developed systems for analyzing the form of utterances in spontaneous language samples. Her Developmental Sentence Types (DST) procedure analyzes utterances which do not contain a subject and verb, that is, are not complete sentences. The DST provides a system for describing presentence utterances that are common in early stages of language development. Lee's Developmental Sentence Scoring (DSS) analyzes utterances that include a subject and verb, that is, are complete sentences. The DSS presents a developmental sequence for personal pronouns, indefinite pronouns, main verb elaborations, negative forms, conjunctions, interrogative reversals, and wh-question forms. Lee proposes remediation plans based on the sequence in which these forms are learned in normal language development. Tyack and Gottsleben (1974) present a procedure for analyzing the use of function words, morphological inflections, and basic sentence constructions in spontaneous language samples. Their analysis results in placing a child at a particular linguistic level of development. Remediation goals are determined by identifying the linguistic forms that a particular child does not use but is expected to know at his or her linguistic level. Miller (1981) presents a system for extensive analysis of language form in children's free-speech samples. The major syntactic categories he analyzes are the fourteen grammatical morphemes identified by Brown (1973) as early-learned, active affirmative declarative sentences, negatives, yes-no questions, wh-questions, and complex sentences that include embedding and conjoining. Miller provides procedures for analyzing simple sentences so that the child's stage of structural development in each category is revealed. He proposes using the child's stage of structural development to establish goals for remediation of syntactic deficits. Klee and Paul (1981) compare six procedures used for analyzing language structure. They describe each procedure and give a comparison of the information gained from each. Persons engaged in analyzing the language of children will find their presentation instructive.

Structured Assessment Procedures Structured procedures often are used for assessing child language. These procedures establish contexts that are likely to elicit particular types of language behavior. The nature and degree of structure imposed varies from general instructions, such as asking the child to tell a story about a picture, to explicit directions to repeat a verbal stimulus. Structured procedures include both nonstandardized and standardized assessment techniques.

Nonstandardized structured tasks have been devised to focus on various aspects of language behavior. Bloom and Lahey (1978) and Miller (1981) discuss the use of elicited responses in the assessment process. Snyder (1975, 1978) devised a set of structured tasks to elicit declarative and imperative functions during activities involving young children. Dale (1980) proposed a slight modification in Snyder's procedures for eliciting the same functions. Berko (1958) designed a procedure for eliciting grammatical morphemes in a structured task in which the child was asked to complete a sentence with a nonsense word associated with a picture. MacDonald and Nickols (1974) present a language assessment instrument designed to elicit utterances that encode certain content categories.

Standardized tests generally are presented in highly structured contexts, since most include specific instructions for administration. Most standardized tests of language content are intended to examine vocabulary. The Peabody Picture Vocabulary Test (Dunn 1965) tests receptive vocabulary. One portion of the Stanford-Binet Intelligence Test (Terman and Merrill 1960) and a subtest of the McCarthy Scales of Children's Abilities (McCarthy 1974) measure expressive vocabulary. The Boehm Test of Basic Concepts (Boehm 1971) is a comprehensive measure of words and concepts that are used frequently in instructions given to kindergarten and first grade children. Its application is with children in the specified age range. Certain subtests of the Porch Index of Communicative Abilities (Porch 1974) evaluate the child's ability to use complete sentences to describe the function of objects, to name objects, to understand and to respond to verbal commands, and to imitate verbalizations of another person.

Numerous standardized tests of language form are available. The Test of Auditory Comprehension of Language (Carrow 1973) is intended to evaluate children's comprehension of syntactic and morphological structures. The Grammatic Closure subtest of the Illinois Test of Psycholinguistic Abilities (Kirk, McCarthy, and Kirk 1968) is a sentence completion task designed to examine children's productive use of certain grammatical morphemes. The Carrow Elicited Language Inventory (Carrow 1974) is a sentence repetition procedure devised to measure children's productive control of grammar.

The specific standardized tests mentioned are but a few of the many available for assessing various aspects of children's language. Most standardized tests are norm-referenced, yielding an age score, percentile rank, or standard score which compares the child's performance on that particular test with the performance of other children. As was stated previously, results of such tests are more useful for identifying the presence of a problem than for planning remediation goals and procedures. The author has found that standardized or other highly structured assessment procedures may be useful to supplement information gained from parents, observations of the child, and analyses of free-speech samples. Rarely do they provide a comprehensive picture of any aspect of child language, and they should not be used as the sole approach to language assessment.

SUMMARY

Children learn to use language to represent their concepts and to convey their intentions. Their learning of language content and form appears to be related to the purposes which they perceive language to serve. They are motivated to learn language so that they can express their intentions in a manner that will reduce the probability of misinterpretation by other people and so that they can organize and learn about their world more effectively.

Studies of normal language learning have suggested predictable patterns of children's acquisition of language use, content, and form. Prior to the onset of speech, infants learn behaviors that signal their intentions as well as systematic routines for interacting with other people. These prelinguistic achievements are the precursors to language. Children's first words encode the intentions that they previously signaled through gestures and vocalizations. The words learned first are determined largely by the intentions that they can be used to express. Children learn which elements in their environment need to be represented linguistically and in what form they should be expressed in order for the intended meaning to be transmitted. With age, normally developing children learn to use language for a wide range of purposes and to engage in conversation following rules and employing strategies that govern appropriate and effective dialogue.

Orderly patterns of learning to represent conceptual content linguistically have been found through studying normal language acquisition. Children learn, through their interactions with others, to use words to refer to perceptible phenomena in their surroundings and then to represent feelings, ideas, and concepts that are not observable. They also learn to encode relational concepts and propositions through combining words. With maturation and additional experience in using language, they learn the linguistic structures that encode major propositional meanings and that modulate the basic meanings of sentences. Throughout the language-learning process, they move systematically toward mastery of the linguistic system of their community.

Some children fail to learn language normally. They may not learn to use language to accomplish an appropriate range of purposes or to engage effectively and acceptably in conversation. For some children, language content may be the primary area of deficiency. They may not learn to use language to refer to people, objects, actions, attributes, feelings, and needs, or they may have difficulty expressing propositional meanings. Others may not learn the linguistic structures which are appropriate for expressing intentions and encoding various aspects of content. Children whose language is deficient in use, content, or form are candidates for language intervention programs. Persons responsible for remediation programs can use their knowledge of normal learning of language use, content, and form in determining the intervention content and strategies that will meet the needs of a language-disordered child.

Assessment is an important part of language intervention programs. Procedures and tools for assessment should be selected on the basis of their utility in assisting the clinician in describing the child's usual patterns of language behavior. Frequently, the most useful procedure is to observe the child in various communication situations and to analyze his or her use of language under different conditions. Information from parents and results of structured tests can provide additional information that contributes to a complete description of the child's language. The results of assessment should provide guidance in setting goals and selecting strategies for intervention.

THREE

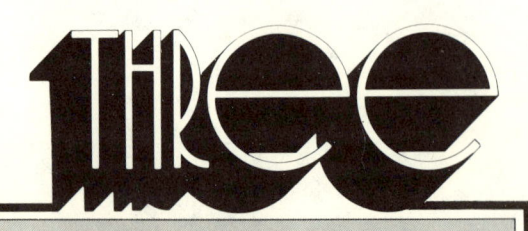

- THE STRUCTURE OF INTERVENTION EXPERIENCES
  - child-centered activities
  - group or individual scheduling
  - physical arrangements
- INTERVENTION PLANS AND PROCEDURES
  - children with limited interactional skills
  - language use
  - summary of intervention for language use
  - language content
  - summary of intervention for language content
  - language form
  - summary of intervention for language form
- SUMMARY

Remediation of language disorders in preschool children

Three

Preschool children with language disorders are entered into remediation programs because their language is deficient in content, form, and/or use. The primary goal of intervention is for children to learn to use language for effective communication. From experiences in intervention programs, children should recognize and employ language as a tool for interacting with other people, for representing themselves both to themselves and to others; for organizing, learning about, and representing their world; and for exchanging ideas and information with others. Their communication experiences should teach them to use linguistic forms for encoding appropriate content to accomplish the purposes for which normally-developing children use language.

Having had limited success in utilizing language for effective communication and learning, many children with language disorders do not consider language to be of value. Their experiences in the remediation setting will influence the conclusions they draw about language and its relevance in their lives. What conclusions do we want children to draw about language from their experiences in intervention programs? They should find that language assists them in accomplishing certain purposes which they consider important. Among the conclusions children should draw are the following:

> Through language, they can influence what other people do.
>
> They can use language to get what they want and to reject what they do not want.
>
> They can use language to call attention to what they find interesting or important.
>
> Through language, they can represent their needs, desires, and ideas.
>
> Their use of language facilitates establishment and maintenance of interpersonal relationships.
>
> Language assists them in gaining new information, in sharing prior experiences, and in making projections about the future.
>
> They can use language to resolve conflicts, defend their viewpoints, and protect their own interests.
>
> Through interpreting what others say, they can benefit from another person's experiences and gain insights into someone else's ideas and feelings.

We want children with language disorders to realize that language serves important functions and that what they say as well as when and how they say it influences their communicative effectiveness. Children's conclusions arise from their experiences in using language. They learn that the content and form of what they say and hear others say, coupled with the context of utterances, determine how they decide what others mean and how others interpret what they say. Through efforts to communicate more effectively and efficiently, they are motivated and guided to learn the language system of their community.

○ THE STRUCTURE OF INTERVENTION EXPERIENCES

Assuming that children's experiences in remediation programs influence their conclusions about what language is, what it is used for, and how it can be used effectively, the structure of remediation experiences takes on great significance. Clinicians need to consider the nature of activities, whether to schedule children in groups or individually, and physical arrangements.

child-centered activities

Intervention programs emphasizing that language is a functional system which is an important part of human experiences are built around children's interests, needs, and abilities. Language is included as a part of their activities. It is incorporated into events so that it facilitates their interactions with other people, their communication of needs and interests, their learning about the world, and their representation of objects, events, ideas, and feelings which are important to them.

In contrast to these language intervention programs, which focus on children's interests and needs and incorporate language into their activities, certain approaches impose language on children with little apparent regard for its utility or relevance to them. Some procedures probably suggest to children that language is an array of lexical items, a series of sentences of a particular linguistic structure, a list of descriptive phrases, or a group of questions and answers, all bound to a limited set of conditions that are, at best, uncommon in their daily activities. The following examples of remediation activities, most of which will not be foreign to people who have been engaged in language remediation for very long, are likely to suggest to a child that language is something other than a useful tool for communicating with someone else about important things:

EXAMPLE A: *Goal*—The child will name x number of objects when shown pictures of these objects. *Situation*—The child sits at a table opposite the clinician, with either the child or the clinician holding a stack of pictures. *Procedure*—The clinician asks, "What is this?" as the child is shown a picture. The child is expected to respond either by naming the pictured item or by using a sentence such as "This is a *(item)*." *Consequence of successful response*—The child is given a star after providing the appropriate answer, and they move to the next picture.

EXAMPLE B: *Goal*—The child will state the action represented in x number of pictures. *Situation*—The child sits facing the clinician, one of them holding a stack of pictures of people or animals engaging in some action. *Procedure*—The clinician shows a picture to the child and asks, "What is the boy (horse, etc.) doing?" The child is to respond either by naming the action or by saying the sentence, "The boy is *(action)*." *Consequence of appropriate response*—The clinician states "Good" or "That's right," and they proceed to the next picture.

EXAMPLE C: *Goal*—The child will use "in," "on," and "under" to identify the location of particular objects. *Situation*—The child sits face-to-face with the clinician, who either places objects in, on, or under another object, or presents pictures of objects in these arrangements. *Procedure*—After placing an object in a certain relationship with another object or showing a stimulus picture, the clinician asks "Where is the *(item)*?" The child is expected to respond either by saying "In (on, under) the table (box, etc.) or "The *(item)* is in (on, under) the table (box, etc.)." *Consequence of appropriate response*—The child is allowed to drop a bead in a box and is given a toy when a specified number of beads have been accumulated.

EXAMPLE D: *Goal*—The child will use the plural marker /s/ or /z/ correctly to mark nouns referring to more than one item. *Situation*—The child and clinician sit on the floor and the clinician shows the child a picture of two (three, or four) items and asks, "What do you see?" The child is expected to respond either by saying "two (three, four) balls (pigs, etc.)" or "I see two (three, four) balls (pigs, etc.)." *Consequence of appropriate response*—The child is praised by the clinician, and they continue with the next picture.

From situations depicted in each of these examples, what conclusions are children likely to draw about language? Probably they would conclude that language is a list of words or a set of sentences spoken in a context in which children find themselves only during the remediation session. As children play, eat, go places, and interact socially with their family and friends, they are unlikely to engage in the types of activities described above. They probably find little relationship between their experiences with language in such sessions and their communicative needs in the rest of their world. Frequently children can be persuaded to participate in such activities either because they like sugar-coated cereal or gold stars, or because clinicians are bigger than children and represent authority figures whose demands, however meaningless or irrelevant, are to be obeyed. However, application of language learned under conditions such as those described in these examples is likely to be reduced because children have not learned to use language as a part of their ordinary activities. They have not been given cause to believe that what they are learning is relevant to their everyday activities.

Instead of engaging children in stilted verbal routines, clinicians can follow the child's lead in finding situations into which language is to be incorporated. As children play with toys, interact with others, encounter obstacles they cannot overcome, make new discoveries, become angry or frustrated, want things they cannot locate or reach, and otherwise act on and interact with their world, the clinician can assist them in learning the language that logically fits into their activities. When children have particular language deficits, the clinician can guide them into situations which call for specific language content, form, and use. The clinician can manipulate the situation so that the target linguistic and communicative behaviors are an important part of the child's activities, thereby making the learning of such behaviors pertinent to the interests and needs of the child. Suggestions for intervention provided later in this chapter show how language teaching can be incorporated into the child's meaningful activities.

group or individual scheduling

Intervention sessions organized around the child's interests and activities can include either groups of children or a single child and a clinician. The author usually finds it more effective to have more than one child participating, provided that the children have progressed in communication development to a point where they show some interest in interpersonal interactions. Certain types of interactions are more likely to occur among children than between a child and an adult. In dealing with another child, children issue demands, engage in arguments, make accommodations, and invite joint activities that may not be a natural part of their interactions with adults. At times other children can be used as models for the target language behavior. An adult can participate with a particular language-disordered child as a partner with the same perspective when one child attempts to communicate with another.

Circumstances may dictate that a child be seen individually rather than with other children, even when a group situation seems more desirable. Time constraints for scheduling, physical facilities, the availability of other children comparable in age or level of functioning, or similar considerations may make individual scheduling necessary. In such instances, the clinician often will have to assume a child's role as a coparticipant in activities and arrange interactions with persons not generally a part of the intervention session (secretaries, other clinicians, persons in the waiting room, custodians, and so on) in order to provide some important types of communicative interactions. However, child-centered language activities can and should be arranged in programs where children are seen individually.

For children who show no inclination to interact with other people, individual scheduling may be most appropriate. Clinicians then are free to react to the child's unintentional behaviors, which can be used to establish joint attention or activity. They can respond immediately to the child's interests, assume both the child's and the adult's role in interactional episodes when such is necessary, and arrange or produce stimuli which are appealing to that particular child. A one-to-one situation may be best when the adult must assume primary responsibility for establishing or maintaining contact and interactions with the child.

physical arrangements

A wide range of physical facilities can accommodate child-centered intervention programs. In order for children to have the opportunity to act, interact, and react with a variety of objects and people under different circumstances, they need space to move around in rather than a confined area, such as that afforded by a small table and chairs or a cubicle. The space available may be small, limiting the size of the groups which can use it with ease, or it may be quite large, requiring that portions be sectioned off to discourage children from isolating themselves in some removed part of the room. Provided that the room is large enough for the children to move from place to place in playing with toys and with each other, the size of the physical space can be utilized effectively by the clinician who selects equipment, arranges furniture, and controls group size carefully.

No prescribed or elaborate set of equipment is necessary in order for a language intervention program to be effective. The primary considerations in selecting materials are that they will be of interest to children and that they are items which the children can manipulate or act on directly. At least some of the materials should be mobile or portable; some should be items whose condition the children can change (paint, cut, eat, and so on); some should be instruments which the child utilizes in accomplishing certain acts (crayons, spoons, scissors, and so on). The items should be capable of entering into different types of relationships with other objects and people —that is, performing actions, being acted upon, changing locations. Clinicians should select materials so that they have a high interest value for the children and so that their use will provide opportunities for the language experiences the child needs to have.

○ INTERVENTION PLANS AND PROCEDURES

Recognizing that children's chief motivation and purpose in learning language is communication, the language intervention plans and strategies described in the remainder of this chapter emphasize assisting children in learning to use the linguistic code to transmit information and bring about results that they find important. The discussion of remediation addresses the aspects of language brought up in the previous section on normal development. A substantial portion of the discussion is devoted to intervention procedures aimed at improving language use, that is, the pragmatics of language. Teaching content and form should be undertaken as a part of teaching language use. References will be given for intervention plans and procedures focusing on teaching content and form.

Readers should keep in mind that the suggested intervention goals and strategies are based on the author's philosophy of language, language acquisition, and the purpose of language remediation. The suggestions for intervention arise from the contention that following patterns of normal development is desirable whenever possible and that children learn language best when it is used in situations that are important and meaningful to them. In the following discussion, there is mention of "instructing," "coaching," or "telling" children to say certain things. When these terms are used, it is intended that the adult will model for children the linguistic forms desired, acting as an assistant or facilitator rather than a drillmaster who has them repeat some word or phrase in rote fashion. In the procedures suggested, the adult should assist children in communicating effectively and not test their ability to repeat what is said or to learn to use memorized utterances in stimulus-bound activities.

Plans and procedures for intervention are given for children who need to learn prelinguistic communicative skills which are precursors to language. The rest of the discussion suggests ways to teach the use, form, and content of linguistic acts. Since there will be variations among children in the specific order of acquisition of language and in types and extent of language deficiency, the areas to be emphasized in any remediation plan will have to be determined according to the needs of each child. Clinicians should select the procedures that are appropriate for a particular child and add to, modify, or discard suggestions according to the child's strengths and deficits.

The suggested procedures presented in the following discussion are intended for children whose primary means of communication will be the use of a conventional linguistic system. Procedures most appropriate for those who need to learn alternate systems of communication are not presented. Readers are encouraged to consult other sources for information concerning programs for children who need to learn nonoral or nonlinguistic means for communicating.

children with limited interactional skills

For children who are not demonstrating social behaviors with which language can be integrated naturally, remediation programs should enhance their learning to interact and communicate with other people. The following suggestions begin with approaches for working with children who do not interact with other people, then proceed to a point at which children express a variety of intentions through nonlinguistic signals. Obviously the appropriate point of entry for any child must be determined by the nature of her or his interactions and communication with other people. The suggested progression toward a readiness to use linguistic symbols communicatively is based on information about prelinguistic communicative development in normal children discussed in Chapter Two. The activities mentioned in this discussion are only examples of possible strategies for guiding the child's acquisition of interactional skills.

Prelinguistically, children develop interactional behaviors through sharing their experiences and activities with other people (Bruner 1978; Lewis 1978; Stark 1978). Their early actions are not intended to signal meanings, but they provide a basis for subsequent learning of intentional communicative acts. Infants first learn an "interaction mode" of behavior. From their social experiences with persons in their world, they learn that they can accomplish certain purposes through their actions. They begin to act with the expectation of getting a response and then with the purpose of signaling a variety of specific intents. This is identified as the "demand mode" of behavior. As they have experiences in exercising control over persons in their environment, children learn the "exchange mode" for interacting. They recognize that other people initiate actions, that interchanges follow certain sequences and procedures, and that reciprocal encounters with others are governed by certain rules. The following discussion suggests plans and strategies to assist children in learning the interaction mode, demand mode, and exchange mode of interaction. Figure 3–1 provides a summary of achievements that are part of these modes of interaction and that form the basic structure for remediation procedures. These are not independent modes of behavior, and the proposed sequence does not imply that there are discrete steps in development. The interactional behaviors in the initial phases are an integral part of more advanced communicative acts, and those

INTERACTION MODE OF BEHAVIOR
    Attention sharing
    Interactional episodes
    Coactions
    Alternate actions
    Routine procedures for interacting

DEMAND MODE OF BEHAVIOR
    Response expectancy
    Intentional acts
    Differentiating acts
    Expanded variety of intentions

EXCHANGE MODE OF BEHAVIOR
    Exchange routines
    Reciprocal interactions
    Conventional signals

FIGURE 3–1 Prelinguistic Modes of Behavior Underlying Language

behaviors that are a part of the demand mode continue into subsequent stages of development.

Interaction Mode of Behavior For children who do not share experiences with other people, intervention should begin with efforts to establish the interactional mode of behavior. *Attention sharing* is necessary in order for interpersonal or communicative interactions to occur. With children who show limited interest in joint-focus with another person, adults need to initiate episodes in which they share the child's line of regard or focus. Initially, the adult should follow the child's lead in establishing a point of mutual attention. The child's own movements or self-stimulating activities may be of greatest interest to him or her and therefore be the appropriate focal point. Objects that move, have contrasting colors, or produce a noise may attract the child's attention and provide a source of mutual regard. Older children may have special interests in a particular toy, pet, noise, or pattern of movement which can serve as a point of shared attention. Once the child's attention is focused, adults should show the child that the item is of mutual interest. This may be demonstrated by touching, talking about, or manipulating an object, or by reacting to a noise or event. Joint focus on an object or event is a prerequisite to social interaction, linguistic reference, and linguistic deixis, and must be established before more advanced interactional and communicative acts can be learned.

Interactional episodes between children and adults contribute to children's learning to share experiences. Adults may need to be persistent in efforts to draw a child's attention toward themselves. Eye contact, exaggerated facial expressions, vocalizations varying in pitch and loudness, head and body movements, or physical contact such as hugging or stroking may call the young child's attention to another person. For children who show an interest in certain objects but not in interpersonal interactions, an adult should participate in activities involving those favorite objects in order to become a part of the children's experiences with items they like. For example, if a child is attentive to a mobile, an adult can activate the mobile while the child is looking at it. If a child enjoys rocking, adults can either hold the child or rock a chair in which the child is sitting, positioning themselves so that the child associates the rocking movement with the actions of the adult. The child's attention to vocal and nonvocal behaviors of another person provides a basis for coactions and alternate action routines, for recognition that other people initiate actions, and for subsequent interpretation of another's communicative acts.

Coactions provide opportunities for children to share experiences with another person. Initially, adults may need to enter into children's activities in order to establish coactions. An adult can join children in their line of visual pursuit, in vocalizing, in facial expressions and body movements, or in posturing. If children engage in routines such as pouring water from one container to another, pushing toy vehicles around the room while producing a vocal sound, or hitting one object with another, adults can become involved in these activities by doing whatever the children are doing. After the children notice that the adult is sharing in the activity, the adult can initiate certain actions taken from the children's repertoire and encourage them to join the activity. For example, if a child has shown pleasure when the adult covocalized or joined in pouring sand from cup to cup, the adult might initiate this activity, encouraging the child to join in. These experiences provide children opportunities to be part of social interactions which they have initiated and which have been initiated by someone else, establishing a basis for later learning of exchange and reciprocal communicative acts. Coactions most often occur during high-arousal states and therefore should be initiated when children are alert and relatively active rather than when they are in a mid-arousal or lethargic state.

Coactions can be transformed into *alternate action sequences*, first taking the form of child-adult-child-adult interchanges. In establishing alternate routines, adults may first need to imitate an act immediately after the child has performed it. The topics for alternate action routines may begin with acts that have been experienced formerly as coactions. Rather than joining the child in producing a vocal sound while pushing the car, the adult may wait until the child pauses in that activity and then perform it immediately. If a child does not take his or her turn in the alternate action sequence, adults may need to assume the child's role as well as their own until the child begins to participate in turn. As the child begins to respond in turn, the adult can shift more responsibility to the child for maintaining the action sequence. Once the child participates in the alternate sequence when the adult imitates an act the child has just performed, the adult can initiate the episode by performing an act that is known to be in the child's repertoire, even when it has not just been performed by the child. For example, if hitting one object with another is an activity which the child and the adult have carried out when it was initiated by the child, the adult can begin an alternate sequence by hitting an object, waiting for the child's response, then hitting the object again. This sets up an adult-child-adult-child sequence of interaction in which the child learns to participate in a social event initiated by someone else. Such experiences provide a basis for subsequent imitative acts and a framework for alternate exchanges in dialogue.

Coactions and alternate actions provide opportunities for children to learn certain *routine procedures for interacting* with another person. These interactional occasions can be organized into play routines in which certain behaviors are used to initiate, interrupt, and terminate interactions. Eye contact, head movements, vocalizing, facial expressions, and physical proximity can be used to regulate the progress of the interaction. For example, eye contact may regulate covocalizing. When either the child or the adult breaks eye contact, the adult also ceases vocalizing and begins again only when eye contact is restored. Turning the head or body can be used in a similar manner to regulate the exchange. This provides children opportunities to learn that either they or another person can exercise control over the flow of interaction sequences and that adjustments in one's behavior may be necessary to accommodate changes in the other's behavior. The ability to alter actions to meet the needs of a social partner is a necessary component of dialogue at subsequent stages of language. The behaviors which are employed to regulate prelinguistic social interchanges are similar to those later used to control conversational exchanges.

Conventional nonverbal acts (for example, pointing) and verbal signals (for example, "look") can be used to expose the child to the relationship between nonverbal and verbal indicators of reference. When looking toward or pointing to an object or event, adults can say "Look" or "There" as part of signaling line of regard. Children's recognition of signals indicating another's line of attention is necessary in order for them to learn to make reference verbally, to use linguistic structures indicating person and place deixis, and to interpret the intent of another person's signals. Recognizing someone else's point of view also provides a basis for later acquisition of conversational rules.

Demand Mode of Behavior Children learn the demand mode of interacting on the basis of their experiences in earlier interactional episodes. They learn to *expect a response* to their actions from occasions in which what they do brings about a noticeable reaction from another person. Initially children may not act with the intent of bringing about a response from someone else. It is important for an adult to respond immediately to children's unintentional acts so that they learn to associate their actions with the subsequent act of an adult. For example, when children wave their arms, an adult may pick them up so that they learn that arm waving brings about this response. When children cry or otherwise vocalize, they may conclude that this causes an adult to come to them if someone consistently responds in this manner. When children knock over or spill something, the adult may respond with exaggerated alarm, using vocalizations, facial expressions, or body movements that children find interesting, thereby indicating that events such as these cause adults to respond. Accompanying responses to children's actions with consistent vocal or verbal expressions provides them experiences in associating vocal patterns or words with acts. For example, the adult may say "up" when picking up a child, "hi" when going to the child in response to vocalizing, or "uh-oh" when responding to the child's knocking over or spilling something. Through such experiences, children learn that verbalizations occur as a part of nonverbal actions.

As children realize that their behaviors bring about responses, they begin to initiate *intentional actions* in an effort to cause something to happen. They learn that the nature of their acts determines the response, and they begin to *act differentially* to achieve more certain outcomes. An adult can assist children by gradually requiring that they respond in a certain way to specific actions the adult introduces as well as by responding in a particular manner to specific actions which children initiate. For example, adults may pick up a child when his or her arms are extended toward them, where before they picked up the child in response to any movement toward them. In playing peekaboo, adults may expose their face only when the child vocalizes, while they previously proceeded with the game if the child vocalized, pulled at the object covering their face, or touched them. The child's nonverbal acts performed with the intent of bringing about certain results are the forerunners of illocutionary force in speech acts.

From successful experiences in bringing about a response to intentional communicative actions, children learn to *accomplish a greater variety of purposes* through their acts. The instumental, regulatory, interactional, personal, and heuristic functions (described in Chapter Two) are among those learned early. Their acquisition can be encouraged in remediation programs. At times when children have material needs or desires, they may unintentionally vocalize or gesture. For example, they may extend their hand toward a cup when thirsty, vocalize as they try to reach a toy, or look from the toy they want to an adult as though attempting to determine whether the adult shares their line of regard. While children may not perform these acts with the intention of causing someone to fulfill their wants or needs, they can learn to use them to accomplish their purpose if the adult responds as though the child's acts were intentional efforts to bring about this result. If children reach toward a cup of milk, hand it to them. If they look from an adult to a toy that is out of their reach, give them the toy. Through such experiences, children learn that their actions can function to satisfy their material needs and desires, that is, to serve an *instrumental function*.

The responses of an adult to children's acts also assist them in learning to use certain behaviors to serve the *regulatory function*, that is, to control the behaviors of particular individuals. Children can learn that by looking at an individual, they signal that they want that person to do something. To assist them in learning this, the individual at whom they look should be the one who responds. If two or more adults come into the room and a child reaches toward one of them, that individual should be the one who responds. While initially children may not move toward either person selectively, they can learn that this behavior signals that they want a response from a particular person if they experience this response on a frequent basis. If the mother consistently responds when children babble "mama," they learn that this particular act increases the probability that they will bring about the appearance of or a response from mother. If a person moves toward or starts to pick up the child and the child turns away, the person's not carrying through with the action will assist the child in learning that by turning away, he or she can reject the actions of another individual, causing them to cease an activity.

Episodes which encourage children to interact with another person were discussed earlier. Some suggestions to assist them in learning to act with the intention of instigating, prolonging, or terminating an interactional episode were provided as procedures for interacting. A number of additional behaviors also are used often for the purpose of interacting with someone else, thereby serving an *interactional function*. Setting up situations in the remediation session so that behaviors serve to establish or maintain interactions will be helpful to children in learning to act for this purpose. Behaviors which establish contact with another person or entice someone else into an activity serve an interactional function. Various forms of greetings (waving, smiling, and vocal gestures) usually bring about a response from the person to whom they are directed. By initiating such behaviors to engage children in interactions or by entering into social games with them when they perform such acts, an adult can guide children toward learning that smiling, waving, or vocalizing can be used to establish contact with other persons or cause them to join in an activity. Similarly, if adults interact with or join the child in a play activity when the child hands them a toy, pulls on their hand, or produces some certain vocal sound, the child will be led to conclude that these behaviors establish interactions with another person.

Prelinguistically, children learn that certain behaviors signal their own feelings, attitudes, or interests, that is, they learn to perform acts which serve a *personal function*. Modeling vocal and nonvocal acts in the situations of pleasure, surprise, anger, comfort, and so on provides the child with examples of expressions of feelings. Grimacing when tasting something unpleasant or when placing something with an undesirable taste in the child's mouth; exaggerating facial expressions, body movements, or gasping in association with sudden movements or unexpected loud sounds to indicate surprise; saying "mmm" or lip-smacking when tasting something pleasant; and clapping or producing a distinctive vocalization during moments of excitement can be used to express one's feelings or attitudes. Children may unintentionally grimace or produce a coughing sound when tasting something they do not like, or they may give a startle response in which they gasp, open their eyes widely, and vocalize in reaction to an unexpected event. If adults imitate, perhaps with exaggeration, children's unintentional reactions immediately after they occur and subsequently use like behaviors under similar conditions, children may come to use these with the intent of signaling their own attitudes, feelings, or interests.

The *heuristic function* becomes more prevalent after the child has begun using language to communicate. However, certain prelinguistic behaviors provide a basis for its expression through language. Children may learn nonverbal acts which assist them in exploring and organizing their environment, thereby serving the heuristic function. For example, they may learn how to work a new toy by handing it to a person who will show them how to use it. By holding a toy up to someone and looking at the person with an inquisitive expression, they can cause that person to name it, show them how it works, or to place it in its logical position. Screaming, throwing a toy across the room, or hitting one toy with another are acts that get someone to provide information that is of assistance in understanding a novel item or experience. In intervention programs, an adult can assist children in learning behaviors that help them in exploring or organizing their world both by responding to the children's requests for help and by demonstrating ways in which children can figure out the use of new objects.

Exchange Mode of Behavior As children learn to express a greater variety of intentions through more discriminating actions, the demand mode of interaction expands into the exchange mode. Certain types of activities within a remediation program can be used to encourage development of this new mode of interaction. In simple *exchange routines,* one person gives another something, the second person returns it to the giver, and this sequence is repeated. Rolling a ball back and forth, taking turns slapping hands with someone else, or handing an object back and forth are give-and-take routines in which the child learns role reversal, first serving as initiator then as recipient of an action. This serves as a basis for subsequent learning of semantic roles and of conversation routines.

Simple exchange routines are transformed into *reciprocal interactions* in which the child and another person have complementary but nonidentical roles in activities which are goal oriented. Reciprocal interactions involve events in which each participant assumes a role, takes a turn, and has a defined task which is regulated by the prescribed actions of the other participant. Within a remediation environment, interactions which encourage the child to learn this mode of behavior might include building a tower, with the child picking up a block and handing it to the adult, who adds it to the tower; picking up toys, where the adult holds open a bag and the child drops toys into it; the adult's holding a doll while the child pulls and releases the string, causing the toy to produce a sound. These simple reciprocal games can be expanded to include more elaborate actions by each participant. For example, in playing with toy animals, the adult's role may be to pick up one of the animals, pretend that it is walking across the floor toward the child, and then hand it to the child, whose role it is to place the toy in the barn. The child may pick up an object and hold it to the adult's mouth; the adult takes it, pretends to taste it, and hands it back to the child, who places it in a box. In washing hands or toy dishes, the child holds his or her hand or the dish under the faucet; the adult turns on the water; the child puts soap on the item; together they rub the object; the adult rinses it.

In teaching children to participate in reciprocal interactions, events should require them to assume certain responsibilities and to rely on another person to take another role in a goal-oriented task. They should learn to anticipate and await a particular act from another person and to fulfill their own role contingent upon the other person's actions. These are behaviors that are important in conversational exchanges and that provide a framework into which children later incorporate language.

Exchange routines and reciprocal interactions provide situations in which the child can learn to use *conventional linguistic symbols* to mark certain aspects of reciprocal interactions. The adult can point to the person whose turn it is, for example, and say "Your turn" or "My turn." The giving of an object can be accompanied by performatives such as *here*, and receiving by *thank you*. Pretending to taste an object can be preceded by *eat* or followed by a comment such as *good!* to signal the completion of that portion of the game. Dropping a toy into a sack held open by someone else can be accompanied by *bye-bye* or *all gone*. Readiness to begin can be marked by clapping, or saying "Okay" or "Ready."

For children who interact socially in the ways described, language can be integrated into their social routines so that it is meaningful. Words become parts of intentional acts, and their use should increase the effectiveness of children's attempts to communicate. So that language will be a meaningful part of what children do, words should be introduced as a part of interesting and important events in the children's world. The use of verbal symbols should facilitate the child's accomplishing the purposes that he or she has attempted to accomplish prelinguistically.

language use

As was discussed in Chapter Two, children learn to use language for certain purposes in different situations. Through their experiences in prelinguistic stages of development and during the course of language acquisition, they learn that language serves a variety of purposes. An important aspect of learning to use language is the acquisition of conversational skills that permit one to engage in verbal interchanges with other people. Language remediation programs can assist children in learning to use language effectively.

Encoding Intentions Children should express a variety of intents through what they say. Those with language disorders may not recognize the range of purposes they can accomplish through use of language, or they may not know how to express their intents linguistically. Intervention strategies can be organized to emphasize the child's use of language for the types of purposes which language serves for normally developing children (discussed in Chapter Two). If Billy uses language as a means of establishing

Another child who expresses a desire for an object by verbalizing can be used as a model, showing the one for whom the lesson is intended that the friend's use of language has positive results. Procedures such as those described in the preceding paragraph can be carried out with several children participating, allowing those who use language for indicating their desires to model the successful use of language for this purpose. An adult can act as a partner to the language-disordered children as they express their desires for items. The adult can coach these children in what to say to get the intended message across to the other children.

Using linguistic forms other than labels for the desired objects can be taught as a means of obtaining what one wants. If children simply name an item in an apparent effort to ask for it, the adult can say "Yes, I see the_____" or "There's the _____," responding to the children's act as though it were intended to call attention to a particular item rather than as a request or demand for it. Providing children with a linguistic form for indicating that they want an object (in contrast to directing attention to it) may be done through use of words such as *Gimme* or *Want,* or phrases such as *Get the*_____ or *Gimme*_____. Use of such words and phrases can be modeled either by the adult or by another child, requiring the language-disordered children to encode the request linguistically as soon as they are able.

REQUESTS FOR SERVICES. Intervention strategies can focus on teaching children to use language for expressing a desire for particular services. If children enjoy being held, rocked, or having their back rubbed or hair brushed, a linguistic symbol can be used to request such services. *Up* may be associated with being held when used either in conjunction with the children's nonverbal gesture indicating they want to be held, or to signal this desire without the gesture. If the child extends his or her arms toward an adult (assuming this is the child's means of indicating a desire to be held), the adult can say "Up" and then pick up the child. Using other children to model the successful use of the word to achieve the intended results may be instructive to those for whom the lesson is intended. Responding to the nonlinguistic gesture in a manner other than that intended by children (shaking the child's hand, as though raising the arms was a greeting; imitating the gesture, as though it was an invitation to enter into a game of mimic) should signal that the intended message has not been conveyed through their nonverbal actions. The addition of the word *up* to the nonlinguistic act should receive the intended response so that children recognize that their use of linguistic symbols increases the effectiveness of their communicative efforts.

Children who encode intents other than a desire for goods and services can learn that words or phrases which accomplish another purpose also can be used under some circumstances to get something they want. If children say "Car" to call attention to an object or to describe an ongoing event involving a car, their use of this word can be responded to as a request for the object. It can be modeled and its utterance required when children gesture to indicate that they want a car. If children say "Ride bike" or "Dolly up" in describing activities they observe or perform, their utterance of these phrases can be answered as though they were requests to perform the activities, or can be required when the children indicate an interest in riding the bike or in having the doll placed in a certain location.

The linguistic forms children are expected to use for expressing a desire for an item or service will vary according to the child's level of linguistic development. If they use single words such as *Gimme* or *Ball* but no combinations of such words, the phrase *Gimme ball* can be modeled and required before the intended response is given. Their use of the single word can be responded to as though its intent were not recognized, thereby motivating them to find another means to express their desires in a more effective way. If they use "Brush hair" to request or demand a service, the importance of more specificity in expression can be demonstrated by misinterpretation of the intended meaning. Rather than brushing the children's hair (if this is the response they seek when they say "Brush hair"), adults can respond by brushing their own or the doll's hair. This focuses attention on the importance of stating whose hair is to be brushed. If children are unable to modify the utterance to resolve the difficulty in interpretation, the appropriate linguistic means of expression can be provided by the adult.

Some children with language disorders express their wishes or needs through linguistic forms that do not readily suggest their intentions. For example, one child said "I ate all my food" to indicate that she wanted to leave the room, even though eating and food were not a part of the immediate context or event. (The clinician and the mother concluded that this utterance as a request to leave was learned because the child was permitted to leave the table at home when she had eaten all of her food.) Another child's utterance of "Daddy's so hot" was his way of asking for something to drink. (His mother proposed that the child associated this utterance with obtaining something to drink because she had used this or a similar phrase on recent occasions when the child's father had come in from working in the yard and she handed him a beverage and said "Daddy's so hot.") These children's use of linguistic forms, however nonstandard, to request items or desires indicates their recognition that they could use language for the purpose of obtaining something they wanted. Appreciating the importance of the continued use of utterances for this purpose, such requests from children should be granted until they learn more conventional forms of expression. To teach more interpretable means of making such requests, responses to the child's statements can be preceded by a word or phrase which represents the intended content. For example, if "I ate all my food" is used to indicate a desire to leave, the adult can say "Go," "Want to go," "(child's name) wants to go," "You want to leave," or "Let's go," and follow this by permitting the child to leave the room. If *Daddy's so hot* is the child's expression for requesting something to drink, the adult can say "(child's name) is thirsty," "I want some water," or a similar phrase that is more appropriate for making the intended request. The author's experience has been that children who use phrases in which the propositional content is not related to the nature of the request often do not use gestures or other systematic nonlinguistic means of expressing desires. When this is the case, it is appropriate to use nonlinguistic signals in association with the utterance to request or state the desire. For example, with *I want to go,* simultaneous gesturing toward the door may be encouraged.

Language to Interact with Others

Children use communicative acts to regulate what other people do, to establish and maintain interpersonal relationships, and to provide information to other people. Those with language disorders may not use language for these purposes, either because they are not aware that their actions can serve these functions or because they do not know how to express these intents linguistically. Intervention programs can be organized so that language-disordered children are provided frequent occasions to express these intents in contexts where their attempts are reinforced. Various means of using language to interact with others can be modeled and the children's efforts modified so that they are more effective and conventional.

REGULATING OTHERS. Intervention strategies can emphasize the use of language to regulate the actions and behavior of particular persons. Adults can demonstrate language to signal who is to do what, sometimes using gestures such as pointing, nodding, or eye contact in conjunction with the verbal signal. For example, contrasting who is to do one thing and who is to do another can be a key part of the remediation events. *John, pick up the toys; Bill, go get the books* can be used with emphasis on the person designated to perform a particular act. Children may be permitted to decide and indicate who will get a certain toy, carry out an activity, assume some designated responsibility, sit in a particular chair, or take the next turn in a game. In these episodes, the emphasis is on use of language to control another individual, to indicate *who* with the result of having that person respond.

In learning to act for the purpose of controlling another person, children may begin by pointing to the designated individual. The adult may ask a child "Who will pour the juice?" allowing the child to select and point to the person who will perform this duty. In conjunction with the child's pointing, the adult can say on the child's behalf "Bill, pour the juice." Once children have learned some means such as pointing to indicate who is to perform the action, the adult can encourage them to say the person's name and subsequently to use more specific verbal symbols to indicate what the person is to do. Through modeling an appropriate linguistic form of expression and encouraging the child to use it, the adult can assist the child in learning a more effective means of telling someone else what to do. The adult can tell children to say "Pour" as they hand the bottle of juice to another child. They can be encouraged to say "Color" as they give another child a crayon with the intention that the other child color a picture.

Games can be structured so that one child is responsible for telling others to perform certain actions. The adult can model and then tell the child serving as leader what to say in such activities, providing the child with repeated opportunities to tell others what to do, with the result of their doing it. The teacher can point to Bill and say "Jump!" to Peggy and say "Sit down," to Max and say "Turn around." The child who then assumes the responsibility of leader can be coached by the adult, with the adult assuming whatever part of leader's role the child cannot handle independently. Similar games can be played with dolls or animals. The child can tell the doll or animal to do something (*Jump, Lay down, Eat, Cry*), and the adult can put the doll or animal through the motions of performing the act.

Demanding that a particular person cease an action or not enter into an event or act are important ways of controlling what other people do. If Kathy knocks over a tower that Rachel is building, the adult can encourage Rachel to tell Kathy "Stop that!" or "Go away!" If Bill tries to take a toy from John, the adult can coach John to say "Don't do that!" or "Stop!" If Larry is about to color on Tom's picture, the adult can suggest that Tom say to Larry "That's mine!" (meaning "Don't touch it!"). If Carrie starts to pick up the dolls that Ron is playing with, the adult can tell Ron to say "I'm playing with those!" (meaning "Don't take them!"). Utilizing the happenings that are important to the child at the moment, adults can assist children in learning a variety of direct and indirect means of using language to demand that another person cease acting in some particular way.

Once children have learned to use language to control someone else in events in which they are involved within the intervention situation, the adult can encourage them to go outside of the immediate situation to ask or tell someone to do something. They can be sent to ask their mother to come into the classroom, to tell another person to turn down the record player, to ask the secretary to open a jar, or to request that another adult sharpen their pencil. If the children's means of requesting is such that their intent may be misinterpreted by the person they are to address, that person may need to be advised in advance so that the experience will be successful. It may be necessary to tell the child how to phrase the request: "Go get your mother. Say, 'Come here, mother.' " or "Go ask Martha to sharpen your pencil. Say, 'Sharpen,' and hold out your pencil like this" (demonstrate to child how to hold out pencil). The form of the request will vary according to the child's abilities and the nature of the relationship between the child and the person to whom the request is addressed. If the child is to use a particular linguistic form (such as *Sharpen pencil* rather than *Sharpen,* or *Open this, please* rather than *Open*), the person to whom the request is made should be aware of the expected form and of the appropriate way to respond should the child use some other means of requesting.

In addition to requesting or demanding, children can learn to use language to control other people's behavior in other ways. Warnings may be issued with the intention of having someone move from a particular place or cease a certain activity. If another child is in the path where Linda is riding her tricycle or pushing a toy car, she may say "Watch out!" or "I'm about to hit you," intending for the other child to respond by moving. If John sees another child starting to pick up a cup that is hot, he may say "That's hot!" meaning "Don't touch it or it will burn you." Within intervention settings, adults can assist children in learning to express and interpret warnings such as these as the need arises during the course of their activities. Acts intended to comfort another person may be used as a means of controlling what someone else is doing. If Jane is crying because she is hurt, Ben can be encouraged to hug her or to say "It's all right now" or "Don't cry anymore." If Joe cries or withdraws from a game because a loud noise frightened him, Bonnie may be told "Tell Joe not to cry. The loud noise is gone." Adults can assist children in using other means of controlling the behavior of another person. These may include bribing (*I'll give you a cookie if you'll_____*), threatening (*I'll hit you if you do that!*), or begging (*Please sing. Please!*). The nature of the request or demand will be determined by the situation and the relationship with the person to whom it is directed. By providing a variety of situations in which children have cause to use language for controlling other people, intervention procedures can give language-disordered children direct experiences for learning linguistic means of regulating another person's behavior.

FACILITATING SOCIAL RELATIONSHIPS. The use of attention-getting acts is an early-learned procedure for engaging others in interactional episodes. Linguistic forms such as *Look, Hey,* or calling the name of a person can be modeled during remediation activities. Adults may use these forms, sometimes in conjunction with nonverbal acts intended to accomplish the same purpose (waving, touching), as they participate in activities with the child or attempt to include the child in what they are doing. Children can be encouraged (or required, if it is certain that the behavior is in their repertoire) to use a conventionally recognized utterance to get someone's attention. The adult can have the child call other people by name to get them to come to a certain location. For example, Sally can call James's name to invite him to join in a game. Or, the child can go to another room to show an item of interest to an adult with whom it has been prearranged that the child must use a linguistic signal to get the person's attention before the adult acknowledges his or her presence. The adult will look up and respond to the child only after the child has said "Look," called the adult's name, or used some other utterance to attract the adult's attention.

Children can be assisted in learning other ways of asking or inviting someone else to join them. Phrases such as *Help me* may be effective in bringing another person into an activity. (This phrase also might be used to get what one wants under certain circumstances.) When a child is attempting to get another to join in a game or activity, the adult can suggest that the child say "Come on," or "Play with me," or can assign the child some role in the activity by saying "You hold the doll. I'll brush her hair." If the child shows an interest in having someone share in looking at a book, the adult may assist the child in saying to the person "Look at this book" or "Read" as they hold the book toward the other person. If one child wants another to play with a particular item, he or she might offer the friend the item, saying "You want this?"

Some children are interested observers of the activities of others but seem unable to inject themselves into the activity. Adults can suggest that these children say to the others "I want to play" or "Can I have a turn?" If other children are playing with particular items or engaging in some interesting activity, the adult can demonstrate to the child ways to join in the game or to enter into the activity by creating a role for himself or herself. For example, if children are playing with a service station, the adult might suggest that the child take a car to the service station and say "I want gas." If children are playing with a grocery store, the child might be told to ask the clerk for some corn or milk.

Young children establish and maintain interactional episodes through use of nonsensical or taunting forms of communication. They may push another child and start running away, attempting to induce the child into a game of chase. They may say in sing-song fashion "You can't catch me" and start moving away from the person to whom they are speaking. They may engage in alternate vocal routines, making meaningless vocal noises. For children who do not participate in such episodes, the adult can go with them into the interactions, taking their vocal or verbal role or prompting the child in the appropriate means of acting to initiate or maintain the interaction.

Children must be responsive to other people's social advances in order to prolong the interaction. Some children with language disorders may not recognize actions of another child as an effort to interact, or they may not know how to respond to encourage continuation of the social exchange. An adult may need to point out to language-disordered children that another child wants them to take part in an activity or is indicating an interest in joining in on what they are doing. If a child walks over to Jack, who is loading animals into a truck, and says "That looks like fun," "I like animals," or simply stands and watches what Jack is doing, the adult may need to point out to him that his friend wants to join him in playing. The adult may say "Jack, Sara is watching you. Maybe she wants to play with you." The adult then can either invite Sara to join Jack or suggest that Jack say "Come play with me" or that he share the animals with her. If a child makes a teasing remark to Jack (*You can't catch me!* or *I can run faster!*) and then moves away as though inviting Jack to play, the adult may need to explain to Jack that the other child wants him to play chase. When language-disordered children do not respond to another person's efforts to engage them in interactions, the adult may need to say "Let's play" and then act in their role to model a means for responding. Gradually, the responsibility for making an appropriate response can be shifted to the child. For a while the adult may need to participate as a partner with the language-disordered child, at first assuming the child's role, then giving the child direct suggestions about how to respond, and finally withdrawing as the child learns to act appropriately in his or her own behalf.

Because conversation is used for the purpose of social interaction, it is important that language-disordered children learn to acknowledge the statements or comments of others as a means of signaling their continuing participation in the interchange. At three to four years of age, children learning language normally begin expecting those to whom they are speaking to acknowledge their remarks. Children with language disorders likely will be left out of dialogic exchanges with their peers if they do not learn how to play an appropriate role in maintaining conversations. Intervention procedures for assisting children in learning to participate appropriately in conversation are discussed later in this chapter.

INFORMING OTHER PEOPLE. Adults frequently use language to provide other people with novel information, and children learn that language can serve this purpose. Intervention programs should assist language-disordered children in learning to use language to inform. Since this is not the predominant function of language for young children, it should not receive excessive emphasis. Children learn to use language to seek new information before they use it extensively to provide others with new information. Language does not serve an informative function unless it represents information that is not known to the addressee. In order to recognize what is unknown and thus informative to listeners, children must be able to assume another person's perspective. Until at least three to four years of age, children with normal language development rarely take into account a listener's prior knowledge and experience and therefore are as likely to encode shared as novel information in their statements to other people.

In intervention procedures, the adult can let children provide others with new information by encouraging them to respond to inquiries from someone else. If a child asks "What's that?" or "Where is the fire engine?" the adult can encourage or assist another child in providing the information. The adult may comment "Billy doesn't know where the fire engine is. Sally, tell him where it is." Such comments may point out to Sally that she is providing Billy with information which he does not have.

Since young children most often talk about the immediate environment, their first experiences in volunteering new information usually refer to an activity in which they have just participated or a condition they have just observed but one which excluded the person to whom they are speaking. In intervention activities, the adult can direct one child to tell another about something the first child has just done but which is unknown to the second. For example, Betty can be coached to say "I painted this picture" as she shows a picture she has just completed to Jack, who has been playing across the room. If another adult enters the room, Peggy can be directed to point to the house she built and say to the adult "I made this house." The child can take something he or she has made to another room and tell someone who made it, how it was made, or some other bit of relevant information that is unknown to that person.

Adults can prompt the child to tell parents or other people who were not participants in the intervention session something that happened during the session. With language-disordered children who do not use language to inform, it may be necessary to be quite specific in prompting (*Tell Mommy what Rachel broke* or *Tell Daddy what you had to drink*) rather than to make general suggestions (*Tell Mommy what we did* or *Tell Daddy what happened*). If the child is unable or refuses to provide the information, the adult can give it on the child's behalf, demonstrating the use of language for this purpose. As the child's ability to report new information improves, prompting and assistance from the adult can be decreased. Likewise, the degree of detail in information to be reported and the linguistic form in which it is to be given can be altered according to the child's abilities and to the context of the utterance.

As children learn to use language to provide information related to times and locations other than the present, they at first are likely to report on conditions or events that involve them directly. In intervention proceedings, they can be encouraged to report on things they have at home. For example, when the child is playing with a truck, the adult can comment "I have a truck at home. Do you?" If the child has been to the circus recently, the adult might engage the child in play with circus animals and then ask if he or she saw a particular animal at the circus, should the child not report this spontaneously. If the child's mother recently has taken an airplane trip, the adult might involve the child in playing with toy airplanes and then ask who rides on airplanes, comment on an airplane trip, or even ask the child if his or her mother rode on an airplane. The extent of direct prompting necessary to get the child to provide the information will depend on his or her ability and willingness to respond.

Language to Observe and Explore the World

Children use language to structure and investigate their environment. In Halliday's classification system (1977), language employed for this purpose first serves a heuristic function and subsequently a mathetic and an ideational function (see Chapter Two). Some children with disordered language experience difficulties in using language for observing and exploring their surroundings. Facilitating their learning of these aspects of language use can be the focus of intervention programs.

OBSERVING THE ENVIRONMENT. Learning to represent objects, actions, and relations linguistically allows children to comment on phenomena they experience and to recall and predict experiences. Young children learn to label objects, actions, and attributes and to represent events and conditions through word combinations. In intervention experiences, adults can demonstrate and encourage the use of language as a means of observing and commenting on items and events that are central to children's activities.

Adults can name objects and actions as they or the children perform certain routine acts. In getting out or putting away toys, setting up art activities, arranging furniture in the doll house, playing with the farm set, or putting pieces in puzzles, adults can name the items or describe the actions that are taking place. The complexity and detail of the comments can vary according to the linguistic abilities of the children. For example, in playing with dolls in a doll house, it may be appropriate simply to name items of furniture, saying "a bed, a couch, a chair" as one places them in the doll house. Descriptive words recognizing attributes may be used in comments such as *the red chair, the little table, mommy's bed.* Action relations can be commented on through statements such as *I'm putting the bed in the bedroom, Mommy's cooking breakfast,* or *Daddy's kissing the little boy on the cheek.* Adults can talk about their own observations or activities in a self-talk manner, or they can comment on what they observe the child doing.

In addition to using language to observe present conditions or events, adults can comment on immediate-past actions and can forecast the immediate future. Statements such as *I covered her up* after one completes this activity or *Now I will get the napkins* as a prelude to this action demonstrate the use of language to comment on the past and to foretell the future.

The use of language for observing the environment does not necessitate a response from another person. It is not intended to cause someone else to act, to change their behavior, or to enter into a social exchange. Language serving an observer function assists one in focusing his or her attention on pertinent phenomena, in directing one's own actions and attention, and in providing structure for the objects, conditions, and activities in the environment.

EXPLORING THE WORLD. Young children learn to use language to check on the accuracy of their perceptions and conclusions and to seek information they do not have. Remediation experiences can be structured so that language-disordered children are encouraged to use language for these purposes. One of the earliest procedures may be children's asking for the names of objects or people. Adults can model "What's that?" as they play with toys or look at books. They may need to provide the answer to their own question if the child cannot answer. Introducing new items among familiar ones will set up a circumstance in which the child needs to ask for the name of the item. The adult can point out the new item if the child does not notice it, perhaps asking the child for the name of the item and then coaching the child to ask another person for the name. For example, if the item is a giraffe and the child doesn't know its label, the adult can say "I don't know what it's called. Let's ask Tommy." The language-disordered child and the adult can take the giraffe to Tommy, and the adult can either ask "What's this?" or coach the child to ask.

Children can be shown how to use language to seek information other than labels. Asking about function, location, attributes, or causes can be introduced into remediation experiences. Rather than drilling the children in use of question forms seeking information they may already have, procedures for inquiring can be taught under circumstances in which the child finds a need for the information. For example, instead of having children ask an adult or another child about the location of an object which is evident, they can be assisted in inquiring as to the whereabouts of something they want but cannot find. Rather than drilling them in using questions asking for the function of items with which they are familiar, they can be introduced to items whose function they do not know and coached in asking someone else for this new information.

Children use language to confirm their perceptions and conclusions. Intervention procedures can encourage and reinforce such behaviors. The child may hold up an object and label it, to which the adult can respond "Yes, a_____" or "No, that's a_____." If young children do not engage in such acts, adults can model this procedure by selecting items for which the child knows the name and asking the child "Is this a_____?" Adults should use the correct label at some times and the incorrect label at others so that the child takes part in both confirming and correcting the proposals.

Comments other than labeling serve to check on the accuracy of one's conclusions. For example, children may make a descriptive statement about something they hear in an effort to determine if their judgments are accurate. They may say "Baby crying" when they hear something in the hall or "Too big" as they try unsuccessfully to fit a large block into a small box. The adult should respond to children's comments of this nature to reinforce their use of language to confirm their ideas. If children do not use language in this manner, adults can demonstrate its use for this purpose by asking for confirmation of their own speculations. For example, if Billy is crying, the adult may ask "Is Billy hurt?" Upon hearing a crash in the hall, the adult may ask "Did someone break a glass?" After using language for this purpose in addressing the language-disordered child, the adult can then serve as a partner with the child in seeking confirmation from another person. The adult may say "Ask Martha, 'Is that a baby crying?' "

Language to Serve More Than One Purpose

Early in their speaking careers, children use an utterance to accomplish a single purpose. One utterance may be made with the intent of obtaining a desired item. Another may be made with the purpose of engaging someone in social interactions. Still another may be intended to seek information about an unfamiliar item. At first, each utterance has a single intent. Once children have learned to accomplish a given purpose through what they say, they begin to express more than one intent through a single utterance. For example, the child may say "Mommy gimme cookie," intending to obtain a desired item as well as to control the behavior of a specific person. A child may say "Brush my hair" in order to obtain a service as well as to engage the addressee in an interpersonal episode.

In intervention proceedings aimed at teaching a child to use language for new purposes, at first an utterance should be used to express a single intent. Once the child has mastered use of language to accomplish several different purposes, he or she is ready to learn that it is possible to express more than one intent by a single utterance. In planning and implementing intervention strategies, clinicians should attend to the purpose for which an utterance is used. In the activities set up to teach a child to request items or services, utterances used for this purpose should not also include specifications of who is to provide the item or service. The child can be taught later to indicate by a single utterance both the desired object and the particular person who is to provide it, so long as the child already knows how to express each of these intents separately.

Language in Conversation As they near three years of age, children become increasingly more proficient at participating in dialogue, as was discussed in Chapter Two in the section on the development of conversational skills. Children with language disorders may have difficulty with conversation because they have not learned aspects of language use which govern verbal exchanges with another person. They may have failed to learn linguistic procedures which facilitate the flow of conversation. They may not have learned to recognize or to signal what information utterances presuppose to be shared by the speaker and listener. They may not know the system of linguistic deixis which is used to mark the role of conversational participants and those referred to but outside of the conversation, and to indicate place and time relative to the moment of the conversation. Intervention procedures can facilitate children's learning to participate successfully in conversational exchanges.

Maintaining the Flow of Conversation

Because dialogue is an alternate-action activity, children must learn to take turns in speaking in order to be effective conversationalists. In the remediation situation, the adult can set up situations in which more than one person has comments to make and require that each wait his or her turn to talk. Interruptions of another person can be stopped with statements such as *Wait. It's Tom's turn. You can talk next.* Rules for turn taking can be established so that the children learn to monitor what another speaker says in order to determine when it will be their turn. For example, if two children are commenting simultaneously on something they have done, the adult can say "Mary, you tell me two things. Then it will be Jan's turn," or "Bill, let Patty tell me about her puppy. Then you can tell me about yours." When the first child's turn is completed, the adult can give a signal that it is the second child's turn. The signal may be pointing to the child whose turn it is or a more frequently used marker of turn in conversation, such as looking at the child whose turn it is to speak. Adults may need to emphasize to language-disordered children the meaning of signals indicating whose turn it is. They may need to tell the children that they will look at, point to, or nod at the one whose turn it is. Additionally, the adult can coach the child in using similar indicators of turn in group speaking activities. For example, the child may ask a question and then point to or call the name of the person who is to answer.

When language-disordered children address another person, they may not realize that they need to do something to cause that person to notice that he or she is being addressed. Demonstrating the use of gestural signals or calling the person's name to get someone's attention may cause children to recognize ways to insure that the person to whom they speak is aware that the statement or question is being addressed to him or her. If language-disordered children fail to employ procedures to indicate whom they are addressing, the adult can coach them in using such signals. For example, if Leon poses a question to Suzanne, whose back is turned, the adult may need to tell him to touch her or to call her name so she will know he is speaking to her. Some children with language disorders do not acknowledge being addressed, so the speaker does not know whether or not they are attending. If this occurs, the adult may need to tell the child to signal in some way that he or she is listening. This may be done by having the child being addressed look at the speaker, answer with "yes," "hm?," "okay," or whatever verbal comment is appropriate for what has been said. To reinforce this responding behavior, adults should always employ some observable signal to acknowledge when they are addressed.

Some children with language disorders inhibit the flow of conversation because their responses are not related topically to what someone says to them. One procedure for signaling topic maintenance is repetition of part or all of the other speaker's utterance. When a child addresses an adult, the adult may repeat some portion of the child's utterance and follow up with a related response. For example, if the child says to the adult "Where dog?" the adult may respond "The dog? Under the table." When the child makes a statement, the adult may add information to the statement. For example, if the child says "Dog big," the adult may say "The dog is big. And he bites." If children respond to what someone says by giving what appears to be a comment regarding a different topic, the adult can point out that the other speaker was talking about a certain topic and the child's response should address the same topic. For example, if Liz says to Paul "Where is my doll?" and Paul responds "That chair is green," the adult can point out that Liz is talking to him about the doll. If Paul does not then make a comment relevant to Liz's question, the adult can ask Liz to repeat the question and then tell Paul what to say that would be an appropriate response. Games can be established to encourage children to attend to and comment on a shared topic. For example, the procedures of a game might have children taking turns naming foods they like, articles of furniture, items in their room at home, things that dogs do, or games that people play. In an activity such as this, the children must learn to stay on topic across speaking turns. The adult can participate, occasionally mentioning an item or activity that is not on topic so that the children learn to monitor the responses of other people.

If children do not give responses which are linguistically contingent on prior statements in a conversation, intervention strategies can be implemented to encourage this behavior. For example, having children complete an utterance started by another speaker requires that they provide a response that is relevant in both topic and form. For example, if the adult says "I like to eat. . . ." the child must recognize what is required both in content and in structure in order to complete the utterance appropriately. Modeling and encouraging elliptical responses also requires recognition of the relationship between the form of the prior speaker's statement and one's response. Rather than having the child answer or comment in a complete sentence, he or she can be encouraged to respond in an elliptical form which is selected on the basis of the form of the preceding speaker's utterance. For example, if the child asks "Who got my candy?" the adult can respond "Roy did," rather than "Roy got your candy." In response to the statement "I like to paint," the adult can respond "Me too" or "I do, too." If children do not begin using elliptical responses appropriately, the adult can direct them in formulating such comments in answer to what someone says to them.

For children who have difficulty maintaining the flow of conversation, adults can participate as a partner with them as they attempt to engage someone else in dialogue. As a partner, adults can assume some part of the child's role when he or she is unable to continue so that the conversation is not inhibited. The adult also can tell the child what to say to the partner in the conversation so that the child experiences use of various conversational devices to encourage continuation of the verbal exchange.

Presuppositions

Children need to learn to determine what information, relative to what is said, is shared by the speaker and listener if they are to be successful conversationalists. They must learn to select what they say so that the shared or given information provides a meaningful context to which new information is applied. They also must recognize the presupposed information underlying another speaker's utterances if they are to interpret what other people say. Between the ages of three and four years, children learning language normally begin altering what they say in light of the listener's needs and abilities. Prior to this age, they rarely change the form and content of utterances to adapt to the listener's knowledge and perspective about the topic of conversation. Presuppositions as a component of conversation in normal and disordered child language were discussed in Chapter Two. The following suggestions for addressing this aspect of language use in intervention programs are based on premises put forth in that discussion. The suggested strategies are examples of procedures for assisting the child in learning to recognize the shared information necessary for interpreting what someone else says; to make appropriate inquiries to gain this information if they do not understand another's utterances; to adapt their utterances in light of their listener's prior or shared knowledge and of the social context; and to alter their communicative efforts to provide the necessary background information if the listener does not have it or does not recognize the information on which their utterances are based.

USING CONTEXTUAL CLUES. The nonlinguistic context is a major source of shared information for children and adults in conversational episodes and often provides the old or given information to which utterances apply. Relating linguistic to nonlinguistic information can guide the child toward recognizing the relationship between what is stated and the immediate nonlinguistic context. Utterances referring to changing conditions (new information) affecting someone or something within the immediate situation (given or shared information) give the child opportunities to relate new with given information which is not expressed verbally. If the adult holds up a toy horse and states "It's broken," the child must recognize the relationship between the given (horse) and the new (broken) in order to understand the meaning of the statement. Pointing or nodding toward a chair (establishing the given) and stating "It fell down" provides an example of new or unknown information which the speaker wishes to point out in relation to the shared item of reference, which was established by the gesture associated with the statement. In the first of these examples, understanding the statement *It's broken* presupposes that the listener and speaker share the knowledge of the item to which the statement refers. To understand the meaning of *It fell down* in the second example, it is presupposed that they share the knowledge that the statement is made with reference to the chair.

Shared activities provide a common base to which new information in utterances can be related. If the adult and child are playing with modeling clay and one of them says "I need some more," the joint activity points to modeling clay as the shared information which must be recognized in order for the statement to have meaning. If a girl hits a boy and the boy says "Don't do that," the action which he is trying to prevent through uttering this statement is shared knowledge based on a common experience and must be recognized by the girl in order for her to understand the intent of his utterance. Experiences such as one child's hitting another, hugging someone else, combing someone's hair, or building a house with another person can provide a shared context to which utterances can be related.

In the intervention environment, the adult can alter the extent to which direct reference is made to establish the given information which is presupposed by a statement. For children who have difficulty picking out the aspect of the environment to which new information in a statement is related, the old or given information can be established by direct gestures or specific verbal reference. For example, stating "The yellow chair fell down" provides within the utterance the given or shared knowledge (which chair) that was indicated in the earlier example by pointing or nodding. Stating "I need more modeling clay" signals more specifically the old information provided by the joint activity in the earlier example. The point of common reference also can be given in a separate statement which is intended to resolve uncertainty in interpretation of the utterance containing the new information. In *Look at the yellow chair. It fell down,* or *You pushed me. Don't do that,* the first sentence provides information presupposed in the second. Moving from specific to less direct reference to the given information should assist the child in learning to interpret new information in relation to the shared knowledge which may not be stated explicitly.

Strategies to assist children in learning to use the prior linguistic context may be necessary in intervention programs. If this appears to be a problem, use of sequential utterances in which the interpretation of an utterance requires recognition of information provided in prior utterances should be emphasized. Reduction in the amount of pertinent information evident in the nonlinguistic environment may be necessary so that the child will focus on the linguistic context in order to interpret what is said. For example, the adult may say "I need a cup. Go get it," so that the interpretation of the second sentence requires use of information in the first. Nonverbal clues, such as pointing toward the cup, can be eliminated as the child experiences success in interpretation without their use. Similar experiences in interpreting can be provided through situationally related statements, such as *Tommy can't lift that box. Help him carry it,* or *I have some cookies. Do you want one?* For children whose language is more advanced, more complex interutterance relations can serve as the basis for interpretation of meaning. Storytelling in which children take turns telling what would happen next requires that they relate previously stated information to what they will say. This can be done in role playing episodes and in creating stories.

USING KNOWLEDGE OF THE WORLD. Some children with language disorders may not recognize that their general information about conditions in the world provides a background against which utterances can be interpreted. Intervention strategies can be planned to address this type of difficulty. Recognition of implausible statements requires children to compare the meaning of what is said with what they know about their environment. For example, pretending to eat inedible objects (*I'm hungry. I'll eat this block*) or suggesting implausible events (*The table will pour the juice*) can be accompanied by overt nonverbal or verbal signals that the statements are ridiculous (making an unpleasant noise when talking about eating an inedible object, laughing or commenting *That's silly* when suggesting an impossible event). Reductions in the overt signals of implausibility can be used to shift to the child the responsibility for indicating that the presuppositions, which must hold true in order for the statement to be appropriate, are incorrect. Knowledge about the world serves as a basis for interpreting other kinds of statements. Regarding items which are broken easily (eggshells, items made of glass or light wood, and so on), warnings about how to handle the objects can move from *Don't drop the egg or it will break* or *Don't step on the airplane. It will break* to less direct forms, such as *It will break* or *Be gentle with this,* which carries the unspoken advice or warning *Don't drop it.* Children who know that items which are hot will burn them can learn to interpret *This pan is hot* as a warning not to touch it.

With those who do not recognize the relationship between knowledge of conditions in the world and indirect expressions of warning, request, or other intentions, the adult may need to express the intent directly, and gradually use more indirect forms. If certain children in a group recognize the intention of the less direct form, the adult can present the indirect form and ask one of these children to verbalize the implication. For example, the adult might point to a freshly painted wall or object and say "This paint is wet. Patty (who understands the implications of the statement), should we touch it?" Patty will reply "no" and can be questioned to elicit her statement of why they should not touch the wall if she does not explain without prompting. The indirect statement *This paint is wet* can be made again, directing the question about the implications to a child who generally does not interpret indirect statements appropriately. If the child's response suggests a lack of understanding of the implications of the indirect form, the adult can supply the more direct form as an interpretation of the less explicit utterance.

RECOGNIZING IMPLIED PRECONDITIONS. Before suggestions, requests, or demands expressed in some utterances can be implemented, it is necessary for certain other actions to be performed. Speakers presuppose that listeners will recognize and satisfy the conditions prerequisite to carrying out the task suggested in the utterance. Some children with language disorders do not recognize the speaker's presuppositions and find the expressed demand or request confusing or impossible to implement. For example, if adults say "I want you to paint a picture," they expect that five-year-old John will recognize that he must get out the paint, brushes, and paper before he can comply with the request. If John has a language disorder, he may not carry out the intended request because he does not recognize the implied prerequisite actions.

Intervention programs can include strategies aimed at helping the child learn to recognize and satisfy necessary preconditions that are not specifically expressed. Beginning with activities in which the child has participated successfully in the past, the adult can decrease the extent to which steps necessary to satisfy preconditions are stated directly, thereby increasing the demands on the child to recognize the presuppositions on which the utterance is based. If bathing a doll is an enjoyable activity for the child, and the adult wants to suggest that they do this, it may at first be necessary to say to the child "Go get the doll. Take off her clothes. We will give her a bath." If the child is holding the doll but the tub in which the doll is bathed is put away in a cabinet, it may be necessary to tell the child to get the tub from the cabinet and put water in it so they can bathe the doll. Moving toward less specificity, thereby requiring the child to recognize the presuppositions that certain conditions will be met before bathing the doll, the adult can say "Go get the doll so we can bathe her," or less explicity, "Let's bathe the doll." If the child does not act to meet the preconditions that were not stated, the adult can add more specific statements or perform the prerequisite actions, perhaps verbalizing "I'll get the doll first and take off her clothes." A variety of activities can be used to assist the child in learning to recognize and act upon presupposed conditions. If the child wants a favorite book which is on top of a shelf, the adult can direct the child to get a chair, climb up on it, and get the book. Later, the instruction can be less explicit, simply telling the child to get the book. If the child has routinely used a wet cloth to wipe up spilled juice, the adult at first may need to state "Get a cloth. Wet it. Then wipe up the juice." Reducing this to "Wipe up the juice" requires the child to recognize the presuppositions about what is to be done prior to carrying out the action stated explicitly in the adult's utterance.

INTERPRETING INDIRECT REQUESTS. Remediation procedures can focus on assisting language-disordered children in learning to interpret the intended meaning of indirect statements, which are a part of many conversational interactions. In routine situations in which certain conditions are commonplace, adults can integrate indirect forms of requests, demands, or other intentions into interactions with children. If the door usually is shut, it can be left open so that the adult can say "The door is open. Shut it, Jimmy." Subsequently, a less direct form of the request can be stated as "I forgot to shut the door" or "The door is open" so that the child learns that such a statement made under certain circumstances actually is a request or demand to shut the door. Similarly, if Susan is asked to give everyone a cookie and Billy comes into the room after she has completed her task, the adult may at first have to instruct Susan by saying "Give Billy a cookie." By later using an indirect form, such as "Billy didn't get a cookie," Susan can learn that under those or similar conditions, the less direct form actually is a request or a demand. When someone is screaming or banging a drum, *That hurts my ears!* can be used as a less direct form of *Stop making that noise!* The degree of specificity expressed should be varied according to the child's ability to recognize the intent of the indirect form and according to the circumstances. If the child does not respond as intended to less direct utterances, more specificity should be added to statements that later will serve as indirect requests or demands.

ADJUSTING TO SOCIAL CONTEXT. Successful use of language in daily experiences is predicated on one's ability to adapt the form of communicative acts so that they are appropriate in various situations and for different social partners. Children with language disorders may not recognize the need to adjust their means of communicating according to the context, or they may not know how to alter what they say so that it is acceptable and effective under varying conditions. Intervention situations can be arranged so that language-disordered children learn to adapt the form of what they say in light of the social situation. Likewise, they can learn from their experiences in communicative interactions to infer important information about social relationships and circumstances from the nature of language used by other people. For example, they can learn that situations may dictate that one speak more softly or more loudly than normal. They can learn when indirect requests are more effective than direct, or when polite or formal terms are in order. They can learn to interpret and to use nonlinguistic behaviors in association with what is said to recognize or convey pertinent information and to modify their communicative acts on the basis of these factors.

Modifying loudness in adaptation to circumstances is one means of adjusting language use according to social context. Creating situations in which alterations in loudness are called for can be done with relative ease within remediation situations. In playing with dolls or toy animals, whispering while pretending that certain toys are sleeping provides an opportunity for adjusting communicative behaviors to accommodate situational conditions. Games in which telling secrets is a part of the activity also create the need to reduce loudness in speaking. Experiences in appropriate loudness of speaking can be created by having a child call someone who is a considerable distance away or by calling to the child from an adjacent room so that his or her response must be loud enough to be heard. An adult can state the implications of someone's use of abnormally loud or soft speech to call attention to its significance. For example, "Jane is whispering. She's telling Tom a secret," "Billy is talking softly because the baby is asleep," or "Ron is talking loudly so that Karen can hear him in the next room" may assist some language-disordered children in recognizing that certain conditions call for modifications in manner of speaking.

Certain types of communicative acts are associated with anger, fear, frustration, or unrest, and signal the actor's feelings. The significance of yelling, emphatic expressions, gasping, a quavering voice, or speaking in hushed tones should be recognized. For example, the adult may need to point out that Nancy yelled because she was angry, that Fred is crying as he talks because he is frightened, or that Tony made the gasping noise because he was surprised by a certain event. Assisting children in interpreting the implications of such aspects of communication may be necessary in order for them to learn the relationship between circumstance and communicative form.

Altering language according to social relationships and the nature of the interaction can be emphasized in intervention situations. The use of polite forms, such as *please* or *thank you,* often represents the first attempts to select utterances so that they are socially appropriate. Adults can model and encourage or require use of such terms under certain circumstances. Some children do not learn to use indirect request forms to make their utterances appropriate for the context. For example, a child may say "Gimme that!" while taking a toy from someone. The adult can say "You should ask nicely. Say 'May I have that?' " If a child demands that another move out of his path by shouting "Move!" the adult can tell the child to say "You are in my way," perhaps explaining that that is a nicer way to ask someone to move. In shared activities such as when two children are playing with clay, the adult can suggest that the child say "I need more clay" or "I'm out of clay" rather than using a more direct form. When parents or other adults are being addressed, the clinician can model polite forms, such as the use of *thank you* and indirect rather than direct forms, telling the child to use these because they are talking to a grown-up. In the prior discussion of ways to help children learn to interpret indirect requests, examples of procedures were given. The adult can let the language-disordered child assist them in using indirect request forms in addressing another child. For example, the adult might tell the language-disordered child that Bill needs to shut the door and then suggest that the child say "Bill, you forgot to shut the door." Letting the child participate as a partner with the adult in issuing indirect requests may assist him or her in learning to formulate requests in this manner.

With some children, role playing or storytelling can be used effectively for experiences in modifying communicative form according to social context. In playing with dolls or in having the child act in some role, a variety of circumstances can be created so that adjustments in the form and content of language are called for. To focus on the relationship between the situation and appropriate language or other communicative acts, the adult may need to state directly that the circumstance calls for certain language behavior. For example, the adult may play the role of the person of lesser social status and say "Please let me go outside," then comment that she said "please" because she was talking to someone she did not know very well. In telling stories, exaggerations in expressions of anger or politeness can be accompanied by direct explanations of their significance in light of the situation. When children are familiar with the events in their context, they can tell parts of familiar stories which call for alterations in expression due to circumstance or social relationships and status.

Questioning for Clarification

If a listener does not know the meaning of some portion of an utterance or if the presupposed information in an utterance is not clear to the listener, inquiries are necessary in order to establish a common basis for interpretation. Some children with language disorders may not indicate when they do not understand an utterance, or they may not indicate which portion they do not understand. Remediation programs may need to include experiences in which language-disordered children learn to seek clarification of information which the speaker mistakenly assumed the listener had.

During interactions with another child or an adult, children may fail to respond appropriately to a request or demand because they do not know what some key word in the request refers to. If told "Give me some more clay," the child who does not know what clay is needs to signal to the speaker that further explanation is needed. Modeling for children "What is clay?" "Clay?" or "What?" may provide them with a way to indicate their need for specific information. An adult can either ask for the information on the children's behalf or tell them what to say to indicate their need for clarification. If they fail to understand the instruction "Put the trucks in the cabinet" because they do not know the meaning of the word *cabinet*, they can be provided with the question "What's a cabinet?" or "Where?" as a means of gaining the needed information. If told to unlock the door and they don't know the meaning of *unlock,* children can be assisted in asking "What does unlock mean?" or "How?"

Some children may not understand something said to them because they do not recognize some presupposed common point of reference. They can be taught to question if they are unsure of the intended meaning. For example, if told "Put the pictures back where they were," assistance in asking "Where were they?" may be necessary in helping them learn to seek additional information that underlies successful interpretation of the request. To respond to "I want some more," the question "More what?" may bring out the information one needs in order to comply.

Children who do not respond as intended may fail to do so because they do not recognize implied prerequisite actions. Those who do not recognize that the instruction "Clean up the mess" implies that they are to get a rag, wet it, and wipe up the paint need to learn to indicate the reason that they find it impossible to carry out the demand. They may need to say "I don't have a rag" or "No rag" to indicate why they cannot perform the suggested task. When children fail to carry out such a request, an adult can question them to determine why (*What do you need to clean it up?* or *Why can't you clean it up?*). Once the reason is discovered, an adult can assist and encourage them in indicating why they found the request impossible to respond to.

For the person responsible for remediation, discovery of the portion of the verbal stimuli that children do not understand provides the basis for assisting them in learning to seek clarifying information. This may be done through observing the nature of the child's inappropriate response, through posing questions to the child, or through altering the nature of the stimuli and noting what portion had to be changed in order for the child to respond appropriately. Once the confusing or uninterpretable aspects of the stimuli have been identified, various forms of seeking clarification can be modeled —that is, performed on behalf of the child to demonstrate that such acts resolve uncertainty—or proposed directly as procedures for the child to employ to gain the needed information.

Providing Clarification of Intent

When persons make statements which presuppose that listeners have information which in fact they do not have, or if shared knowledge basic to the statement is not evident, it often is necessary for the speaker to alter what they say in order to provide additional information. Some children with language disorders have difficulty restating what they say when it is unclear to or misinterpreted by the listener. When asked for clarification, the child may give no response, repeat what was said originally, or make substantive changes in what was said. Children with language disorders may need assistance in learning to recognize what portions of their utterances need to be clarified for the listener's benefit.

Adults can point out to children whose utterances have not been interpreted correctly the portion of the utterance that was unclear and can model for them ways to restate it. For example, if a child asks another for a knife and is given a napkin, the adult can explain "She doesn't know what a knife is. Tell her, 'The one that cuts.' " If the child says "Hurt me" in a context in which the person who hurt him is not known, the adult can explain "I don't know what you mean. *Who* hurt you?" If no response is given when the child says "Go get the crayons," the adult can explain that the addressee doesn't know where the crayons are. A suggestion such as "Tell him, 'Go get the crayons. They are on the desk' " may provide the child with a useful way to clarify the message. If the child says "Jimmy has a new bike" and the listener does not know who Jimmy is, the listener likely will say "Who's Jimmy?" The child may need assistance in explaining who Jimmy is. Questions such as "Is Jimmy a boy?" or "Is Jimmy your brother?" may be necessary to assist the child in determining what information is pertinent in responding to the question "Who is Jimmy?"

Deixis

The nature of the deictic system in conversation and its acquisition by children was discussed in Chapter Two. Since deictic terms are meaningful only within the conversational context in which they are used, children do not learn them until they have learned to engage in dialogue. Terms which are used to indicate speaker, listener, and those external to the conversation—that is, person deixis—begin to be acquired before other forms of deixis. In English, the principal deictic terms for person are personal pronouns. Some children with language disorders may not learn that first person pronouns refer to the speaker, second person pronouns to those whom the speaker is addressing, and third person pronouns to those not involved in the immediate conversation. Structures marking deixis of place, that is, referring to locations relative to the speaker, generally are not used in a contrastive sense until after three years of age. Children with difficulties in language use may fail to learn terms such as *here, there, come,* and *go* to indicate location relative to the speaker. Linguistic devices marking time of events relative to the time of the utterance, or time deixis, usually are not acquired until after age three. Children's failure to learn lexical items or morphological markers indicating time demonstrate difficulties in learning the system of time deixis. Since linguistic deixis is an important component of discourse, its inclusion in intervention programs is important. Aspects of interaction that are precursors to linguistic deixis as well as use of deictic terms can be a focus of remediation procedures.

Certain distinctions are basic to learning deixis of person, place, and time. Differentiations between one's own and another person's perspective and the ability to make proximal/distal distinctions are prerequisite to learning linguistic forms whose meanings are tied to recognition of the speaker's versus another person's point of view. The prior discussion of intervention procedures for developing prelinguistic communicative skills addressed several aspects of interaction that underlie learning of linguistic deixis (pp. 106–114). These included activities to encourage following another person's line of regard or pursuit, signaling to indicate one's own point of attention, taking turns, role reversal, recognition of temporal sequences of events, and establishing points of reference for specific communicative acts. If children in a language intervention program have not reached a level of communicative maturity to learn the linguistic deictic system, they should be involved in interactions in which they acquire those skills which are prerequisite to learning linguistic deixis.

PERSON DEIXIS. Deixis of person is learned before place and time deixis because appropriate use of person deictic terms requires fewer shifts in reference. First person pronouns always refer to the person speaking, second person pronouns to those being addressed, and third person pronouns to those referred to but not participating in the conversation. First and second person contrasts seem to be simplest to learn because they require only shifting of roles of the speaker and listener. Third person pronouns can refer to anyone not included in the immediate conversation and therefore can have a variety of reference points.

Before using deictic terms to indicate person, children learn proper names as linguistic devices signaling individual identity and differentiating one person from another. Gestures accompanying the use of proper names when referring to self as speaker and to another as listener reinforce the use of communicative acts to point out the participants' roles in dialogic interchanges. Within intervention episodes, adults can model the use of gestures in conjunction with proper names during dialogue. For example, when asking who wants another cookie or who wants to play with the dishes, children can be guided to point to themselves as they say their own name. When addressing other children, the child who is speaking can be guided to point to addressees when referring to them by name. If someone says "Who wants to paint?" the adult can assist Linda in pointing to herself as she says "Linda" or "Linda wants to." Once Linda uses such actions to indicate that she is referring to herself, the adult can tell her to say "I want to" as she points to herself. Having several children in a group refer to themselves as "I" illustrates that this word refers to whoever is speaking and is not just another name for a single individual. Using the above example, each of several children can be coached to say "I want to" or "I do" in response to the question "Who wants to paint?" Use of other forms of first person pronouns also can be incorporated into a variety of activities. For example, "My doll" or "Mine" can be modeled as adults pick up an item and hold it close to them. If Sherry generally refers to herself by name so that she would call a treasured item "Sherry's book," she can be told to tell Ralph "Sherry's book. Mine!" or "My book!" when he attempts to take it away from her. At the end of the period when children are preparing to go home, an adult can hold up coats, art work, or other possessions which the children are to take with them and ask "Whose_____is this?" The expected response from the owner may be "My_____" or "Mine." Such an event in which all children use first person pronouns to refer to themselves as they speak focuses attention on the fact that these forms refer to whoever is speaking.

Intervention strategies can emphasize the use of second person pronouns to indicate the person being addressed. Adults can point to the child whom they are addressing and say "Jack, *you* pick up the blocks," and subsequently omit the child's name, saying "*You* pick up the blocks" while pointing to the child being addressed. A child can be given the responsibility of instructing others to do various things. If needed, the adult can assist in indicating who is to do what, telling the child to point to Bill and say "You get the chalk" and to Sharon, saying "You get the erasers." To contrast first and second person pronouns, adults can point to themselves and say "*I* will get the dishes" and to the child, saying "*You* get the dolls." Adults also can assist a child in telling another "*I* am playing with the animals. *You* play with the clay" or similar types of contrastive statements. Other contrasts between first person and second person forms can be illustrated through statements such as "My coat" and "Your coat" or "Mine" and "Yours." For example, in dividing toys to be played with, adults can say "My block" when placing a block in their stack and "Your block" when giving one to the child. Adults can encourage and, if needed, instruct the children in stating "My animal" (or "Mine") as they place a toy animal in their own stack and "Your animal" (or "Yours") as they give one to the child to whom they are speaking. To show that these deictic terms reflect speaker in contrast to listener, children engaged in activities such as dividing toys can take turns giving out the toys so that all experience using *I* (*my, mine, me*) to refer to themselves and *you* (*your, yours*) to refer to others involved in the incident. With changes in speakers, they experience being referred to with the term *you* (*your, yours*) by another speaker and hearing other speakers refer to themselves using *I* (*my, mine, or me*).

After the contrast of *I* and *you* is used and interpreted meaningfully, the terms *we, us,* and *our* (*ours*) can be introduced in referring to the speaker and listener together. Commenting on joint activities is one way to illustrate that *we* refers to both speaker and listener. For example, the adult can say "*I'll* get some blocks. *You'll* get some blocks. *We both* will get some blocks," pointing to indicate to whom reference is being made. In moving chairs from one place to another, the adult can say "*I'm* moving chairs and *you're* moving chairs. *We're* moving chairs together." Reference to shared possessions can be used to illustrate use of terms such as "our" or "ours." Rather than giving one cookie to the child and another to the adult, they can share a single cookie. The adult can say "This is *your* cookie and *my* cookie. It is *our* cookie. *We* will share it." When a child and adult are coloring a picture together, the adult can say "*We're* coloring this picture together. It is *ours.*"

Within conversational episodes, use of third person pronouns to refer to persons not engaged in the conversation can be contrasted with deictic terms indicating speaker and listener. Initially the distinction can be made more clearly by using *she* (*her, hers*) and *he* (*him, his*) to refer to persons involved in activities clearly separate from those in which the speaker and listener are engaged. For example, when the adult and a child are engaged in a mutual activity such as dressing a doll, the adult can say "*I* will put on her socks. *You* put on her shoes. Beth isn't helping us. *She* is playing in the sand," pointing to Beth, who is in another part of the room. When giving crayons to children who are preparing to color, adults can say as they give one to each child "*You* get a crayon. *You* get a crayon. Tom doesn't need a crayon. *He* is not going to color with us," pointing to Tom, who is engaged in an activity elsewhere. When several children have been engaged in an activity together and one leaves to do something else, adults can say "*I* want to build a house and *you* want to build a house. Sheila doesn't want to. *She* has gone to look at the books." Once children recognize that *she* and *he* refer to persons other than conversation participants, use of *they* (*them, their, theirs*) can be introduced to refer to several people other than those taking part in the conversation. For example, the adult may say to a child "You and I will get out the juice and cups. Paul and Jan are busy. *They* can't help us." When sharing something with a child, the adult can point out "This is *ours*. Mary and Jennifer have one, also. That one is *theirs*," pointing to an item being shared by children not participating in the discussion at the moment.

PLACE DEIXIS. Learning terms for deixis of place is preceded by use of other linguistic forms to indicate proximity relative to self and to others. For example, children can be taught to refer to locations as *by me, near me,* or *close to me* in making reference to the position of objects or actions. Terms such as *beside Jim* or *in your lap* can be used to indicate locations relative to someone else. Deictic gestures pointing to place relative to self and to others also can be a useful prelude to learning linguistic forms for deixis of place. Pointing in conjunction with *by me* to indicate the desired location of an object can be an effective means of signaling location relative to self. Once reference to location, either linguistic or gestured, has been learned, deictic terms indicating location relative to the speaker can be introduced by using them in conjunction with previously learned means of indicating. Proximal terms, such as *here, this,* and *these,* should be taught before distal terms, such as *there, that,* and *those*. Since proximal terms have a more constant reference point, that is, near the speaker, they are easier to learn than distal terms, which can refer to any location away from the speaker.

Initially, adults should use place deictic terms from locations near the child so that their spatial perspective will be the same as the child's. This diagram shows such an arrangement:

Distal item of reference ☐	Proximal item of reference ☐	○ Adult
		○ Child

Sitting beside the child, adults can say "Put it right *here,* close to me," or "The doll is *here,* by me." The term *here,* used under such circumstances, is appropriate from the child's as well as the adult's perspective. Similarly, standing beside the child, adults can say "Pick up *this* block," pointing to the block near them. Adults can coach the child to tell someone else "Sit *here,* by me," or to say "Put the animals in *this* pen, beside me." Distal terms, such as *there, that,* and *those,* also should be used initially from a perspective shared by the child and adult. Accompanying the statement with a gesture, the child can be told "The ball is over *there,* not near us," or "I want *those* blocks. I can't reach them."

Once children begin using and interpreting terms for place deixis with themselves as the point of reference, intervention strategies can be implemented to assist them in learning to recognize the meaning of such terms from another person's point of view. Initially, the perspective of the second member in the conversation should not be directly opposite the child's. In other words, the meaning of the proximal and distal terms should not have to be reversed in order to be used appropriately by the participants in the dialogue. This arrangement should be such that the child and adult do not share the same perspective for proximal terms but do for distal terms, as in the following diagram:

	Item proximal to the child ☐	○ Child
Distal item of reference ☐		
	Item proximal to the adult ☐	○ Adult

Under these circumstances, *there, that,* or *those* would refer to a location away from both the child and the adult, while *here, this,* or *these* would refer back to the speaker, whose perspective is different from the listener's. Children would have to learn that *here, this,* and *these* make reference to locations near the speaker, whether or not the speaker shares their perspective. However, they would not be required to recognize distal terms from a perspective other than their own, since locations distal to them also would be distal to the other person. To assist the child in learning to interpret deictic terms indicating locations proximal to another speaker, the other speaker may use such terms in conjunction with person deictic terms, which the child already should know to interpret from the speaker's viewpoint. For example, the speaker may say "*This* one is *mine,* right *here,*" pointing to a location nearby.

When the child has learned that proximal terms refer to locations near the speaker no matter who or where the speaker is, the child's partner in dialogue can move to a position opposite the child, as shown in the following diagram:

Child ○ □ Item of Reference   Item of Reference □ ○ Adult

With this arrangement, the child will need to learn that distal, like proximal, terms are to be interpreted from the speaker's perspective. What is *here* to the child will be *there* to the adult. Associating deictic terms of place with previously learned markers of person deixis may assist the child in recognizing the necessity of taking the speaker's viewpoint in interpreting the meaning of the terms. In speaking to the child, the adult may say "The dog is *here,* by *me,*" or "The truck is *there,* by *you,* not by *me.*"

While verbs such as *come-go* and *bring-take* are not expected to be used as deictic contrasts until after seven years of age, they can be introduced in association with other deictic terms of place before that time. For example, "Come over here," "Go over there," "Bring it here to me," and "Take that over there to him" may be used to expose the child to the use of such verbs deictically.

TIME DEIXIS. Prior to learning terms which establish time of events or conditions relative to the time of conversation, children learn to refer to the order of events in which they are involved. They may indicate temporal order by stating "My turn," "I'm next," "You go after me," or "First ___ ; then _____." Attention to sequence and its linguistic representation can be the focus of intervention activities. In events where several children are involved, the adult can say "It's Dick's turn now. Then it's Pat's turn" or "Carla will be next." In routine activities which normally occur in a particular sequence, verbalization of the order of activities can be used to demonstrate the linguistic representation of the temporal sequence. The adult can point out "First get out the crayons. Then draw a picture." To involve the child in verbalizing the sequence, the adult can say "It's time for juice. What do we have to do first?" to which the child is to respond "Pick up the toys" (assuming that routinely the toys must be picked up before having juice). If a child spills paint, the adult can say "Peggy, you spilled the paint. What do you do now?" to which Peggy can respond "Wipe it up."

Once children are using linguistic forms to refer to the temporal ordering of events in which they are immediately involved, they can begin learning terms to indicate time other than the present. Upon completion of a task in which the adult and the child participated, the adult can comment "We made a big fence for the animals. That was fun." After a child has finished a project, the adult can refer back to the activity, stating to the child "Tom, you picked up all of the blocks. You did a good job!" "Finished," "all done," or "through" can be used to refer to activities completed prior to the moment of speaking. If a child has built a bridge with blocks and moved on to another activity, the adult can point out "Rachel built a bridge. She's not building it anymore. She's *finished* building the bridge" or "Ted painted this picture. Now he's *through* painting." As in the above examples, initial reference to prior events should be about activities in the recent past and, when possible, about activities which included the child or which the child witnessed.

As children become interested in reporting on events outside of the immediate context (not until at least age four in most children with normal language), words such as *yesterday,* or *last night* or *one time* may be used to indicate a time in the past. To provide a common topic for all children in the group, reference can be made to something that happened earlier in the day or on the previous day. A calendar on which events of each day are indicated can be used to focus on something that the children did the previous day. The adult can comment on the item pictured on the calendar for the previous day or ask the child to do so. The adult may say "Yesterday we made Kool-Aid," or ask a child, "What did we do yesterday?" perhaps pointing to the picture on the calendar to refresh the child's memory. If children take turns performing some task such as picking up the cups after juice time or distributing coats when it is time to leave, the adult can make reference to the person who did the task the previous day. "Who picked up the cups yesterday?" may provide the children opportunity to refer to a past event in which they were involved. Projects can be left unfinished from one day to the next so that there is reason to refer to what was done yesterday. Children's relating of past events not associated with the immediate context (past trips with the family, something that happened to a sibling, what they did over the weekend) may be infrequent until late in the preschool years. When they begin attempting to refer to past activities of this nature, pictures from the event or some item associated with where they went or what they did may assist them in relating the experience.

In learning to represent future events, terms such as *later, in a few minutes, after awhile,* or *not now* can be used to mark times subsequent to the present. To point to events which will occur in the near future as a part of the present context, the adult can say "It's not time for cookies now. We will have cookies later," or "Let's play with the farm set now. We will get out the clay in a few minutes." If a child wants a particular item that someone else is using, the adult can say "Sam is playing with the zoo animals now. You can play with them after awhile." To assist children in learning to use linguistic forms to represent future time, the adult can tell the children something they will do the following day. For example, the adult may say "It's time to go home now. You will come back tommorrow. Tomorrow we will make popcorn." If a project is to be completed the following day, a comment such as "Tomorrow (or next time) when you come back, we will put icing on the cookies."

Some children learn to use grammatical morphemes to mark temporality relative to the time of conversation before they signal such times lexically. Irregular verb forms may be learned most readily, since they are separate lexical items and are more salient perceptually then regular verb inflections. In referring to events that occurred within the present context and the recent past, adults can emphasize use of grammatical forms to refer to the past. Holding up a painting, the adult can ask "Who painted this?" to which the child will be encouraged (coached, if necessary) to reply "I did." Referring to a job just completed, the adult may say "Who finished making this house?" expecting a response such as "Bill did." In playing with dolls, the adult might ask "Is the baby still asleep? No. She *was* sleeping, but now she's awake." If a child comes up with an item that has been lost, the adult can comment "I thought the scissors were lost. Where did you get them?" The child can be encouraged to respond "I found them." Modeling use of the new form, the adult might comment "Look. Sherry found the scissors. They aren't lost anymore." Forms signaling future events can be emphasized in a similar manner. In preparing for an activity, the adult can pose questions which encourage use of forms referring to future acts. When getting ready to bathe a doll, the adult may ask "Who will get the tub?" and then encourage the child to respond "I will."

Marking past time with verb inflections can be encouraged through the manner in which children's utterances are interpreted and through emphasizing the meaning of the inflections. If a child reports to an adult "Tim kick down my house," the adult can point to Tim and say "Tim isn't kicking it now." The child may report "Look," pointing to the shattered house, giving the adult opportunity to say "Your house is already broken. Tim kicked it." A child may run to the adult and say "Sue jump on the furniture." The teacher can ask "Is Sue jumping on it now or has she stopped?" If the child reports that the jumping is no longer going on or the adult sees Sue doing upon, or change states. Their first verbs refer to actions they initiate or are affected by or that cause changes in states of objects. Early-learned attributes express changeable or transitory states of objects rather than permanent conditions. Children learn to combine words to represent relational concepts that they previously signaled through single words in combination with gestures and with the nonverbal context. Their first propositional meanings expressed through word combinations refer to what they do or see others doing, to associations between people and objects, to relations between actions and objects, and to attributes and locations of people, objects, and events. In learning both the referential meanings of single words and the propositional meanings of multiword utterances, young children show a preference for dynamic rather than static conditions. Language is a part of what children are doing, of what is happening in their world. It is not used as a passive description of the static conditions they observe passively.

Intervention programs to assist children in learning the semantic component of language should reflect the notion that language learning is a dynamic process. Strategies adopted should insure that the children learn words as a part of the activities in which they are involved, not as a set of labels for remote objects or actions. The concepts they express linguistically, either as single words or as propositions, should assist them in accomplishing the purposes they wish to accomplish through speaking.

The following discussion of remediation for those with deficiencies in language content emphasizes the types of conceptual information that young children learn to encode linguistically. It addresses children's learning of the referential meanings of words and of propositional meanings encoded through multiword utterances. Teaching language content should be integrated into episodes in which language use is stressed so that the content provides specificity for the pragmatic intents children encode.

Referential Meanings of Words For children who have a limited vocabulary, clinicians must decide which words to teach. Holland (1975) and Lahey and Bloom (1977) present excellent discussions of criteria for choosing a core vocabulary for intervention programs. Based on their suggestions and on information discussed previously relative to normal language development, several guidelines are suggested for selection of lexical items to include in early stages of language learning.

1. Lexical items should refer to entities, actions or processes, and conditions or attributes with which the children are involved frequently.

Nouns should refer to items the children manipulate, to objects and substances they want, and to persons (or other animate beings) they wish to control or interact with. Nouns should stand for objects the children touch, bend, push, pull, stack, throw, eat, break, hit with another object, place in various locations, and encounter in other ways. They should include names of important people and pets with whom the child interacts.

Verbs should refer to actions or processes in which the children frequently engage or to those they want others to perform or to assist them in performing. Verbs should represent actions which the children initiate or are affected by (*run, jump*), those by which they act upon other objects (*break, eat*), and actions which result in changes in location of objects (*fall, throw*). Verbs may include actions which children want another person to perform in their service (*gimme, help*), which call for the attention of another person (*look, come here*), and which control activities of someone else (*stop, sit*).

Attributes should make reference to changing or unusual conditions of objects. They may be conditions the children have caused to change (*broken, all gone*) or states which affect them directly (*hot, dirty*). Attributes also may assist the children in identifying a particular object, creating new labels (*Mommy's book, black cat*) rather than contrasting objects (*red coat, blue coat*). Words representing permanent states (*big, green*) should be introduced when differentiation of objects on the basis of such attributes becomes communicatively significant to the child.

> **2.** Lexical items should refer to objects and events which occur in more than one instance.

Children first learn that a noun, verb, or attribute refers to a single instance and then that the word represents a class of objects, actions, or conditions having certain features in common. So that they will learn that labels represent a category of objects, items should be available in similar but nonidentical forms. The object with which they first identify a word serves as a prototype and therefore should be representative of the general category of objects to which that word normally applies. For example, children are more likely to generalize the word *ball* to represent many different balls if they first learn it in association with a round ball rather than with a football, which is the only ball with an oval shape. Similarly, they learn action words first as representing a particular instance of the action and then to refer to similar actions. It is important that they experience use of the word under different circumstances so that they will realize that it refers to a category of actions. For example, they may first use the word *eat* only to refer to what they do to a cookie. Through hearing *eat* used with reference to what they, other people, or animals do to other edible substances, they learn that *eat* does not simply refer to an action involving a single entity.

3. Words learned initially should represent items at a midlevel of generality, with those designating more specific or more generic classifications being introduced later.

Young children's communicative needs do not require reference to narrowly defined subcategories or to broad, generic classes of items. Labels at a midlevel of generality serve their communicative needs. For example, *cookie* and *sandwich* will suffice, although later they will find cause to differentiate these categories as *chocolate chip cookie* and *peanut butter cookie* or as *cheese sandwich* and *ham sandwich,* and to refer to the more generic class, *food.* *Dog* and *horse* express their intents, and *collie* versus *beagle* or *Shetland pony* versus *palomino* are not significant differentiations to young children. Beginning around age four, normally developing children show an increase in usage of words representing more specific and more generic classifications of items that have been represented previously at a midlevel of generality.

4. Lexical items which can be combined easily to express semantic relations should comprise a significant proportion of a child's vocabulary.

The entities and actions encoded by single words should combine naturally to express semantic relations that are common in children's early two-word utterances. They should represent entities that disappear, are rejected, and reappear, and that initiate and receive the force of actions during the course of children's activities. They should refer to actions and processes that animate beings initiate and that affect the location and condition of entities with which the children have frequent contact. Lexical items should have the potential for use in a number of different phrases which express semantic relations. For example, in expressing the relation agent-action, *mommy* can serve in an agentive role with a number of different verbs, and *go* is an action that can be performed by many different animate beings. In action-object relations, *ball* can serve as the object affected by or receiving the force of many verbs. The combinatorial potential of words should be considered in selecting lexical items to teach.

5. Lexical items that express one's attitudes, feelings, and interests should be included in children's early vocabulary.

In order for language to serve a personal function, children need affective words. These words may have limited combinatorial potential, and they may not refer to tangible items or actions. They provide children with linguistic devices for expressing feelings such as love, excitement, frustration, anger, and fear. These devices may include words such as *hug* and *kiss,* which represent actions expressing positive emotions. They also may include *goodie, yeah,* or *yuk* or a variety of other expressions which at times may be of questionable acceptance socially. The use of such words is important in order for children to learn to represent themselves through language.

The specific lexical items to be taught will vary according to the children's interests and to the home and remediation environment. Some children show a greater interest in trucks, cars, and mechanical toys, while others prefer animals, dolls, and toys representing animate beings. Some enjoy creative activities, such as painting and playing with modeling clay, and others generally choose active games, such as chase or bowling. In the home situation, one child may stay indoors most of the time, helping parents with household chores or coloring, playing with blocks, and watching TV. Another child may spend substantial amounts of time outdoors, helping with yard work, playing on swings, and taking part in group games such as hide-and-seek or kickball. In choosing the lexicon to be emphasized in the intervention program, clinicians should take into consideration the children's preferred and usual activities so that they will have frequent occasion to use the words they learn.

The discussion of normally developing children's patterns of learning lexical items was presented in some detail in Chapter Two. Clinicians are encouraged to consider that information in planning strategies for teaching word meanings to language-disordered children.

Propositional Meanings Children learn to use multiword utterances to encode relational meanings they previously conveyed through combining single-word utterances with relevant nonlinguistic clues available in the immediate context. Some language-disordered children do not learn to express propositional meanings linguistically. They continue to rely on the listener's ability to integrate their one-word utterances with situational information for interpreting what they say. Intervention programs for such children should address teaching the use of multiword utterances to express relational meanings.

The early semantic relations expressed by children learning language normally was discussed in Chapter Two. Figure 3–2 presents the most frequent early-appearing operations of reference and semantic relations as well as those which occur with less frequency in the initial period of multiword utterances. These combinatorial meanings represent relational concepts children have acquired in prior periods of development. They refer to children's perceptions and conclusions about the relationships among people, objects, actions, processes, and states. The semantic relations are the basic elements to be emphasized in intervention programs to teach young children to express propositional meanings.

Clinicians must decide which relations to introduce first. Studies of normal development indicate that most children encode operations of refer-

FIGURE 3-2 CONTENT OF EARLY LINGUISTIC PROPOSITIONS

FREQUENTLY ENCODED RELATIONAL MEANINGS

Operations of Reference

Nomination-existence	There (this, that, the, a) + referential word
	This puppy; That mommy; There book
Recurrence	More ('nother) + referential word
	More milk; More block; More run; 'Nother baby
Nonexistence-disappearance	Allgone (no, no more) + referential word
	Daddy allgone; no car; no more spoon
Rejection	No + referential word
	No juice; No drink
Denial	No + referential word
	No break; no here; no spill

Semantic Relations (two-term)

Agent-action	Daddy jump; Baby hit; Puppy run
Action-object	Hit car; Up baby; Eat cereal
Agent-object	Baby (read) book; Mommy (throw) ball; Daddy (push) bike
Action-location	Go (to the) park; Play outside; Sit (on the) chair
Entity-location	Baby (is in) bathtub; Puppy (is) outside; Shirt (is on) chair
Possessor-possession	Brother('s) truck; Baby ('s) cookie; Daddy ('s) doll
Entity-attribute	Dirty hand; Doll (is) broken; Daddy (is) wet

Semantic Relations (three-term)

Agent-action-object	Baby hit ball; Mommy push bike; Baby read book
Agent-action-location	Daddy go store; Puppy play outside; Baby sit chair
Action-object (possessor-possession)	Eat baby('s) cookie; Put-on mommy('s) hat; Ride brother('s) bike
Action-object (entity-attribute)	Wash dirty hand; Hug wet puppy; Ride red bike
Action-location (possessor-possession)	Sleep daddy('s) bed; Play Jack('s) house; Go baby('s) room
Action-location (entity-attribute)	Ride red car; Go big store; Sit broken chair

RELATIONAL MEANINGS LESS FREQUENT IN STAGE I

Semantic Relations (two-term)

Action-instrument	Cut (with) knife; Draw (with) pencil; Hit (with) hammer
Agent-instrument	Baby (cut with) knife; Mommy (paint with) brush; Daddy (dry with) towel
Action-beneficiary	Give (it to) mommy; Read (the book for) baby; Pour (milk for) baby
Action-comitative	Go (with) daddy; Come (with) mommy; Ride (with) brother

Semantic Relations (three-term)

Agent-action-instrument	Mommy cut (with) scissors; Baby write (with) pen; Brother build (with) hammer
Action-object-beneficiary	Give mommy (the) book; Get candy (for) baby; Read book (to) baby
Agent-action-comitative	Baby go (with) mommy; Brother sing (with) baby; Baby ride (with) daddy

ence before semantic relations between nouns and verbs. Attention to the children's predominant communicative style may provide guidance in choosing the relations to present initially. If a particular child most often uses communicative acts to label or refer to objects and actions (mathetic function), this child may learn most easily to express relational meanings of existence, entity-location, possessor-possession, and entity-attribute. Another child, primarily interested in using language to control or interact with other people (pragmatic function), may learn action relations more readily. By responding to the children's communicative preferences in selecting the relation to introduce first, the adult may insure that the children will find encoding semantic relations to be useful communicatively. However, just as clinicians must plan intervention strategies to teach children to use language for a broad range of purposes, they also must include expressions of all semantic relations as a part of the program. While the children's preferences in communicative style may provide guidance in selecting the semantic relation to teach first, such preferences must not lead to the exclusion of certain semantic relations in the overall intervention program.

The semantic relations which appear first in most children's speech are listed in figure 3-2 as Frequently Encoded Relational Meanings. These express relational concepts which seemingly are most important to young children and therefore should be the first introduced in intervention programs. As children learn to express these relations and to show an understanding of other relational meanings, the less frequently used relations should be included in the program. Those which appear in Stage I speech but with less frequency include instrument, beneficiary, and comitative relations. They are listed in figure 3-2 as Relational Meanings Less Frequent in Stage I.

To teach children to express semantic relations, adults should provide linguistic representations of the activities that children perform, wish to have others perform, or observe with interest as someone else takes part in an activity. They should be presented so that their use facilitates children's expressing pragmatic intents, and a specific semantic relation should not be tied to expression of a single intent. The two-term and three-term relations shown in figure 3-2 can be used to assist children in getting what they want, in controlling other people, in interacting socially, or in commenting on and exploring their surroundings. Operations of reference can be used to express several intents. Expressions of nonexistence or disappearance (*Book allgone*) and of nomination (*There mommy*) might be used to check on the accuracy of one's perceptions (heuristic function) or to establish joint attention (interactional function). Expressions of recurrence (*More milk*) might be used to request items (instrumental function), to call someone's attention to an item (interactional function), or to organize experiences (heuristic function). Rejection (*No truck*) can be used to turn down an item (instrumental function) and, like expressions of denial (*Not break*), to indicate one's own feelings or position (personal function). Relational meanings expressed between nouns and verbs also are used to express a variety of intents. Agent-action relations (*Mommy sit, Daddy read*) can be used to control what a particular person does (regulatory function), to observe or organize the environment (heuristic function), or to call someone else's attention to a situation or event (interpersonal function). Action-object relations (*Hit ball, Get cookie*) and action-location relations (*Sit chair, Go store*) can be used to make a request or demand (instrumental function), to engage someone else in a mutual activity (interactional function), or to observe existing conditions (heuristic function). In similar ways, other relational meanings can be used to assist children in making their intents understood under varying conditions. The expression of relational meanings should be incorporated into activities described in the previous discussion of teaching language use.

In intervention programs for children first learning to encode relational concepts linguistically, semantic relations should be introduced one at a time, that is, several relations should not be introduced simultaneously. Once children have learned to express a relation in several contexts, a second can be introduced, although continued use of the initial relation will receive attention in intervention activities. For example, if the agent-action relation is the first to be emphasized, the adult will model the use of this relation under several conditions in which the children are involved and will assist them in using it as part of their communicative acts. Once the children encode the agent-action relation in several circumstances, a second relation, such as action-object, can be introduced. The children need to be encouraged to extend their use of the agent-action relation to new contexts while they are learning the second relation, action-object.

Once children have learned to express two-term utterances, expansion to three-term utterances should be presented systematically. Expansion occurs in one of two ways. Two-term utterances can be combined and the redundant term omitted, as in the following examples:

```
(Agent – Action) + (Action – Object)      Agent – Action – Object
 Boy      hit        hit       ball         Boy     hit      ball


(Agent – Action) + (Action – Location)    Agent – Action – Location
 Mommy    go         go       store         Mommy    go      store
```

Expansion from two-term to three-term relations also can be accomplished by expanding one constituent so that it becomes a relation. For example, the object in an utterance may be represented by a possessor-possession relation, as in *Wash baby('s) hand* or by an attribute-entity relation, as in *Eat big cookie*. Three-term relations are composed of combinations of earlier-learned two-term relations. Similarly, two-term and three-term relations can be expanded into four-term relations either by concatenation of previously learned relations or by expanding one term so that it is a relation. In teaching children to program more relations into a single utterance, clinicians should follow these systematic patterns of expansion.

Children's ability to encode relational meanings linguistically is dependent on their learning linguistic forms which represent these meanings. They must learn to combine words and to use grammatical morphemes which signal the semantic relations between words in multiword utterances. Intervention programs for language-disordered children should include procedures which assist children in learning to use linguistic structures to convey meanings effectively.

summary of intervention for language content

Since young children show a greater interest in dynamic conditions than in static conditions, the referential and propositional meanings first emphasized in intervention should represent objects, events, and relationships involving actions or changes in states. Lexical items should refer to objects and actions with which the child is involved frequently and in varying contexts. The types of propositional meanings learned first have been documented for normally developing children. Since it appears that the semantic relations encoded first represent young children's concepts about relationships in their world, it is logical that these early-learned semantic relations should be the starting point for teaching language-disordered children to encode propositional meanings. Children learning language normally follow systematic patterns for increasing the number of semantic relations they program into a single utterance. Intervention goals and strategies should follow a similar pattern for assisting language-disordered children in learning to increase the semantic complexity of utterances.

The contexts in which language content is taught should be natural for the child. If children learn to encode referential and propositional meanings as a part of their expressions of pragmatic intents, they are more likely to recognize the importance of learning utterances which represent certain aspects of their experience. They will use words and word combinations more meaningfully and frequently if they learn from experience that this helps them to reduce the probability of misinterpretation of the intentions they wish to express.

language form

The learning of linguistic form cannot be considered separately from the acquisition of the pragmatic and semantic aspects of language, since linguistic structures are devices used to signal pragmatic and semantic meanings. Normal acquisition of linguistic expressions of pragmatic intents and of the conceptual content of utterances was considered in Chapter Two. Earlier in this chapter, the discussion of intervention procedures for children with deficits in language use and language content also included suggestions for teaching children to use various linguistic forms. Those suggestions provide a basis and a format for teaching language form. The discussion of the acquisition of syntax in Chapter Two addressed normal developmental patterns of children as they learn to use language structures to transmit meanings. Those patterns of development provide guidance for persons in charge of intervention programs to assist children in learning to use linguistic structures to convey meanings. The following discussion highlights several considerations that should assist persons in planning intervention strategies to teach language form. These suggestions should be applied to the earlier discussion of the acquisition and teaching of the pragmatics and semantics of language.

The major aspects of language form to be considered are linguistic devices for marking semantic relations, early-learned grammatical morphemes used to modulate the basic meanings of utterances, and several sentence forms learned by young children to express various intents and meanings. For each of these aspects of language form, major points for consideration in setting goals and strategies for remediation are given.

Marking Semantic Relations The first syntactic device which most children learn is the use of word order to signal the semantic relations between words. Later, they learn to use prepositions to indicate some relational meanings. The patterns of normal development discussed in Chapter Two provide guidelines for clinicians as they teach children to mark relational meanings linguistically. In planning strategies for teaching children who are entering the stage of multiword utterances or for those who do not use word order and/or prepositions to signal meanings, the following points should be of assistance.

1. In talking to children and in assisting them in formulating utterances for communicating with other persons, clinicians should structure their utterances so that the linear position indicates the semantic relations between the words.

In young children's utterances, preverbal nouns represent the initiators of action—usually animate beings. Utterances should take the form of *Baby cut* rather than *Scissors cut,* and of *Brother break window* rather than "Rock break window." Objects affected by actions, locations, and instruments are usually inanimate, and words representing these concepts appear postverbally (*Roll bike,* or *Go [to] store,* or *Cut [with] scissors*). Clinicians should adhere to set patterns for ordering words to mark the semantic role of nouns and verbs until children are honoring that order in their utterances.

>   2. When teaching children to program more than two terms into a single utterance, two-term relations already encoded linguistically should be combined or expanded systematically.

Children learn to express three-term and four-term relations either by concatenation of two-term utterances or by expanding one term so that it expresses a relation. This procedure was discussed in Chapter Two and earlier in this chapter. As children learn to expand utterances to include a greater number of semantic relations, word order continues to be used to signal relationships between words.

>   3. Prepositions should be taught according to the semantic relation they mark, not as individual lexical items or as a generic grammatical class of words.

As children have learned to encode relational meanings through word order, they learn to mark some of these relations by prepositions. The order in which children learn prepositions to signal semantic relations was discussed in Chapter Two. Prepositions should be taught according to the relation they mark rather than as separate lexical items marking a variety of relations. For example, *to* should be taught first as an indicator of location (*Run to school*). Subsequently, *to* may be taught in contexts in which it indicates a beneficiary relation (*Give it to Sam*) and to introduce an object complement construction (*I want to play baseball*). Similarly, children should learn *with* to mark comitative relations (*Ride with us*) separate from learning it to signal an instrument relationship (*Write with a pen*).

>   4. Prepositions should be taught to indicate semantic relations which children are already encoding linguistically.

Children encode relational meanings through word order before marking them by prepositions. Before introducing a preposition to signal a relational meaning, clinicians should be certain that the children are expressing that meaning through some other means. For example, the children should be encoding locative relations through word order (*Sit chair*, or *Put blocks box*) before locative prepositions are stressed as markers of relations. Similarly, they should express instrument relations (*Cut knife*, or *Sweep broom*) and beneficiary relations (*Give coat mommy*, or *Buy candy baby*) before prepositions are emphasized to mark these relations.

Grammatical Morphemes to Modulate Meaning Children learn to use grammatical morphemes to modulate basic meanings expressed as semantic relations. Prepositions, which are one kind of grammatical morpheme, have been described as markers of semantic relations. The fourteen grammatical morphemes usually learned first by English-speaking children as well as the order of acquisition and factors which influence their learning were discussed in the previous chapter. That information should guide clinicians in setting goals and planning strategies for teaching language-disordered children to use grammatical morphemes appropriately. The following suggestions point out some of the factors which should be considered in intervention procedures.

1. Grammatical morphemes should express concepts children have already acquired.

New linguistic forms should be taught to encode information or knowledge that the child has. For example, adding plural markers to nouns to signal more-than-one should be emphasized only after the child has indicated an awareness of multiple instances of items. Teaching grammatical morphemes to indicate time prior to the present should occur after the child is making reference to past events. Children should be taught to use the possessive *s* only after they demonstrate an understanding of the relationship between a possessor and a possession. Clinicians should be aware of the meanings signaled by grammatical morphemes and have cause to believe that the child understands these meanings before emphasizing the use of a morpheme in the intervention program.

2. Grammatical morphemes should be taught first in contexts where their presence is necessary in order for their meaning to be conveyed.

In many contexts, grammatical morphemes are semantically redundant. Their meaning often is signaled by lexical items or other linguistic forms within the utterance. For example, the *-ed* on *jumped* is a redundant marker of tense in the utterance *Jack jumped yesterday,* since the word *yesterday* also signals time prior to the present. The plural *s* on *girls* is a redundant indicator of number in the phrase *two girls,* since *two* indicates plurality. In the utterance *The dogs have a doghouse,* the plural *s* on dogs is redundant, since *have* indicates more-than-one when its subject is a noun. The present tense form of the verb *to be* often does not convey additional meanings. Forms of this verb, whether used as a copula or an auxiliary, mark number, person, and tense. Number and person also are signaled by the sentence subject in most utterances, making the verb redundant in these regards.

regards. Unless otherwise indicated, it is assumed that the utterance pertains to the present, and therefore use of the present verb form does not provide new meaning. In order for a *to be* verb to carry a maximum semantic load, it should be taught as a marker of tense in utterances where prior time is not otherwise indicated. This would include utterances such as *Jack was at home*, or *He was running*, or *She was sick*. Plural markers on nouns should be taught in contexts in which the grammatical morpheme is the only marker of plurality (*I want the blocks*, or *The girls ran*, or *He gave me the cookies*).

    3. Grammatical morphemes should be taught in contexts which enhance their perceptual salience.

Perceptual salience appears to be a factor which influences children's learning of grammatical morphemes. This suggests that they should be taught in contexts in which they are most conspicuous. Several factors increase the perceptual salience of grammatical morphemes. In teaching linguistic forms to mark past tense or plurality, irregular forms are more salient than regular forms. For example, the change from *eat* to *ate* is more obvious than the change from *walk* to *walked*. The phonetic substance of grammatical morphemes affects perceptual salience. For example, syllabic plural markers (*houses, roses*) are more perceptible than those represented by a single phoneme (*lips, gates*). The linear position of the grammatical morpheme in the utterance makes it more or less perceptible. Utterance-final forms are more obvious than those embedded within the utterance, so that the plural marker is more likely to be noticed in the utterance *the dogs* than in *The dogs ran*. Teaching irregular before regular forms may call the child's attention to the fact that the meanings carried by a particular form are marked through alterations in word forms. Selecting words whose phonetic structure is such that grammatical morphemes bound to them are syllabic may have a similar effect. Structuring the linguistic context so that morphemes occur in utterance-final positions should assist in calling the child's attention to the target form. For example, teaching possessive *s* or regular past tense forms may be done best through presenting them in elliptical utterances (*Who got that?* or *I did* or *Whose coat is this?* or *Jack's*).

As was noted in the discussion of the normal acquisition of grammatical morphemes, the meaning of the morpheme, its semantic and perceptual salience, and its semantic and grammatical complexity all influence children's learning of these linguistic forms. Each of these factors should be considered in intervention strategies. So that the children will learn to use these structures in normal communicative situations, whenever possible, they should be taught during natural speaking events rather than in routine drills in which language is removed from their reality.

New Sentence Forms Children's early utterances generally are simple declarative sentences. While they may omit sentence subjects, thus producing utterances which would be classified as imperatives in adult language, such sentences should not be considered as imperatives until the child begins using them in an exclusively imperative sense, that is, to demand, request, or suggest. The normal acquisition of various sentence forms was discussed in Chapter Two. Information from that discussion should assist clinicians in organizing remediation procedures for teaching children to use different sentence forms. The following guidelines are suggested for planning intervention strategies for teaching new sentence forms.

1. Variations in sentence forms should be taught as a means of encoding pragmatic intents.

Children learn to select various sentence forms to indicate the nature of their intents in speaking. Negative forms may be used to reject or deny a proposition or to observe or declare something about one's self or the environment. Imperatives are used as a direct means of requesting, demanding, or suggesting actions on the part of another person. Initially, question forms are used to seek confirmation or rejection of one's perceptions and conclusions, and to ask for new information. Later, children learn to use question forms as indirect means of expressing other intents (requesting, demanding, denying, and so on). In teaching children to use sentence forms other than the simple declarative, clinicians should consider the pragmatic intents the new form can express. They should teach alterations in sentence forms in situations where the child has the need or desire to express the intent which the sentence form suggests.

2. The semantic content of the utterance should influence the order and strategies for teaching new sentence forms.

The semantic structure of question forms influences the order of their acquisition. In yes/no questions, all semantic relations are specified, and the respondent is asked to confirm or negate the proposition. In wh-questions, one major semantic constituent is unknown and is represented by the wh-word. Children will not learn question forms in which a word playing a particular semantic role is asked for until they have learned to encode that semantic role in declarative sentences. For example, they will not use or respond to *where* questions appropriately until they have learned to express location in declarative forms. Children learn *who, what,* and *where* questions, which ask for actors, actions, objects, and locations, before they learn *when, how,* and *why* questions, which ask about time, cause, and manner. The nature of information sought by the first wh-question types is less complex than that sought by the latter wh-question types.

In learning to coordinate sentences, children must recognize the semantic equivalence of separate sentences or of sentence constituents. They must learn that sentences which can be coordinated refer to conditions or events that are related temporally and spatially and that sentence constituents must play identical semantic roles in order to be coordinated. To use embedded sentences, children must recognize the relationship between the propositions expressed in the individual sentences. They must realize that one sentence expressing a proposition can serve as a semantic constituent in another, as in object complement constructions (*He likes to play ball,* or *Look at that boy eating ice cream*). In such instances, the proposition in one sentence plays a certain semantic role in relation to the main verb in another sentence. To formulate embedded sentences containing relative clauses, children must recognize that one proposition can provide additional information about a single constituent in another proposition but be unrelated to the basic proposition of the sentence in which it is embedded. For example, in the sentence *I got the pencil that belonged to Jack,* the relative clause *that belonged to Jack* refers to *pencil* but is not a part of the basic noun-verb relations in the sentence *I got the pencil.* Clinicians should keep in mind that children appear to learn to embed propositions that serve a major semantic role in another sentence before they learn to use relative clauses. They also should consider that the semantic complexity of each sentence influences the ease with which children can perform embedding operations. For example, embedding a two-term utterance in a two- or three-term utterance is simpler than embedding a three-term utterance in one that contains a greater number of semantic relations.

> 3. The transformations required to formulate various sentence types should influence clinician's teaching of the forms.

To formulate imperative sentences, children must learn to delete the sentence subject, which refers to the person to whom the sentence is directed. Formulating imperative sentences is not as complex as formulating question forms. To transform *John is here* into *Is John here?* one must perform a transposition operation. In formulating wh-questions, one must prepose the wh-word, which represents the missing constituent, and transpose the sentence subject and the auxiliary verb. These operations change *John is going where* into *Where is John going?*

Children first begin to mark question forms by rising intonation only, producing sentences such as *Daddy is coming home?* In formulating wh-questions, they first learn to prepose the wh-word and produce questions such as *Where he is?* or *What he is doing?* Later they learn to transpose the auxiliary verb and the subject to produce *Where is he?* and *What is he doing?* In teaching children yes/no and wh-question forms, clinicians should be aware of the transformational complexity of utterances, accepting less than perfect constructions during the learning process.

In learning to coordinate sentences and sentence constituents, children must learn to compare the syntactic structure of sentences and sentence constituents. They must recognize that the form of sentence constituents to be coordinated must be identical and that they must play the same grammatical role in their parent sentences. Children must learn to perform deletion transformations as well as to have knowledge of the grammatical structure of sentences in order to perform coordination and embeddings. Clinicians should keep in mind the types of knowledge of linguistic structures that are necessary in order for children to perform coordination and embedding operations.

summary of intervention for language form

Children learn linguistic forms to assist them in expressing pragmatic and semantic meanings. Word order appears to be the first syntactic device they learn to mark semantic relations. For language-disordered children who are just beginning to combine words or who order words unconventionally, clinicians should attend closely to the linear positioning of words in their utterances to the children and in the utterances they assist them in formulating. To teach children to use prepositions to mark semantic relations, the prepositions should be taught according to the semantic relations they signal, not as individual lexical items or as a grammatical class of words.

Studies of normal language learning have indicated which grammatical morphemes children appear to learn first to modulate the major meanings of utterances. Clinicians should teach these in contexts where they carry maximum information load and where their perceptual salience is greatest.

In teaching children to use new sentence forms, clinicians should pay attention to the pragmatic and semantic aspects of meaning to be expressed. From their experiences in the intervention sessions, children should learn not only the syntax of various sentence types but also when it is appropriate to use which sentence forms.

Syntax should be taught, whenever possible, as a device for expressing intentions and concepts. New linguistic forms should be taught to represent concepts which the child has already developed. Rote drills designed to teach syntactic structures should be used only as a last resort.

Summary

Young children who are not learning language normally are entered into language intervention programs with the expectation that under appropriate circumstances, they can improve their ability to use the linguistic system as a mechanism for encoding intentions and concepts. Some children with disordered language may not have acquired the prelinguistic knowledge and skills that are precursors to language learning and use. For such children, intervention plans and strategies should focus on establishing prelinguistic behaviors and abilities that lead to language learning. Some children with deviant language may have a narrow view of the purposes which language can and should serve for them. With these children, intervention strategies should be developed with the intent of helping the child recognize the functions which language can fulfill and teaching him or her how intentions can be verbalized effectively. Language-disordered children may not know how to use language in conversation. They may need programs and procedures that stress learning basic conversational rules and linguistic procedures for participating successfully in conversation. Some language deficits may include difficulties in representing conceptual content linguistically. Children may be deficient in learning the referential meanings of words and/or the propositional meanings of multiword utterances. Intervention programs for these children should include strategies to assist them in learning to use linguistic symbols to stand for phenomena they experience. Many children's language is described as deficient because they have not learned the linguistic forms in which language should appear. They may not learn conventional procedures for combining words to represent their experiences and ideas or to convey their intentions. They may learn to encode basic propositional meanings but not to use the grammatical morphemes that modulate the basic meanings of utterances. Intervention plans for these children should include specific attention to teaching language form. It is the responsibility of those who participate in planning and/or implementing remediation programs to determine the nature of a child's language deficits and to create a program that will address the child's needs.

The suggestions for language remediation presented in this book reflect the author's contention that intervention programs for preschool children with language disorders should follow a development approach to language learning. This means that the program content should be selected and sequenced on the basis of what is known about patterns of normal development. The context in which the intervention program is implemented and the strategies for teaching should be chosen in light of what is known about factors that appear to enhance or inhibit normal language learning. Language-disordered children are unlikely to learn language from occasional or incidental experiences with language. In intervention programs, situations can be set up or manipulated so that a child has frequent and repeated opportunity to use language or to see others use language in ways that will emphasize the aspects of use, content, or form that the child needs to learn.

The recommendations for building language intervention programs around situations of language use reflect the author's contention that language-disordered children, like those developing normally, will be motivated to learn language because of what they find they can do with it. Their learning to use language for a variety of purposes, and their seeking to accomplish their purposes with minimal misinterpretation will cause an interest in learning to express new meanings in conventional linguistic form. It has been the author's experience in working with young children with disordered language that they generalize and apply what they learn within the intervention setting much more quickly and appropriately if they have learned language within a context that provides experiences of importance and interest to them. In other words, emphasizing language use and teaching content and form as a part of activities that are important to the child has brought about better results than teaching content or form isolated from meaningful use and then trying to teach the child how to employ the structures that have been learned when they use language in other settings. Structured drill on some linguistic forms should be used as a last resort and only with children whose language use and content are adequate.

Numerous sources suggesting remediation procedures for language-disordered children are available. L. Miller (1978) describes intervention plans and procedures which are centered around the pragmatic aspects of language. Simon (1980) presents a detailed program in which language use is the basis for teaching language content and form. Readers should consult other sources for developing intervention programs focusing on teaching language content and form, since these were treated only generally in this book. Miller and Yoder (1974) and MacDonald and Blott (1974) give plans and procedures for teaching language content, especially with reference to encoding semantic relations. Stremel and Waryas (1974) provide plans for teaching language form and structure to children with deviant language. Waryas and Stremel-Campbell (1978) discuss procedures for teaching language form in conjunction with language content and use. Lee (1974) details the planning of intervention programs for children whose primary deficit is in learning to use linguistic forms appropriately. *Syntax Two* (Ausberger 1980) is a systematic program for teaching children to use linguistic structures.

Readers are encouraged to consider the theoretical and philosophical bases for proposed language intervention programs (including the suggestions given in this book) before they adopt any procedures. No single program will fit every (or perhaps any) child. Persons who plan and carry out remediation programs should have a well-thought-through philosophy of what comprises language, how children learn language, and the purpose of language remediation. The most exciting, and at times the most frustrating, part of planning and implementing language intervention programs with young children is that an abundance of new information about human communication and its disorders becomes available almost daily. Clinicians should take advantage of new information and alter programs and procedures in light of what is known about child language and breakdowns in language learning.

References

Anglin, J. *Word, object, and conceptual development.* New York: W. W. Norton, 1977.

Aram, D., and J. Nation. Preschool language disorders and subsequent language and academic difficulties. *Journal of Communication Disorders,* 13 (1980), 159–70.

Ausberger, C., *Syntax two.* Tucson, Ariz.: Communication Skill Builders, 1980.

Austin, J. *How to do things with words.* Cambridge, Mass.: Harvard University Press, 1962.

Baltaxe, C., and J. Simmons III. Language in childhood psychosis: A review. *Journal of Speech and Hearing Disorders,* 40 (1975), 439–58.

Bangs, T. *Language and learning disorders of the pre-academic child: With curriculum guide.* New York: Appleton-Century-Crofts, 1968.

Bates, E. Acquisition of pragmatic competence. *Journal of Child Language,* (1974), 277–81.

Bates, E. Pragmatics and sociolinguistics in child language. In D. Morehead and A. Morehead (eds.), *Normal and deficient child language.* Baltimore: University Park Press, 1976, 411–63.

Bates, E., L. Camaioni, and V. Volterra. The acquisition of performatives prior to speech. *Merrill-Palmer Quarterly,* 21 (1975), 205–226.

Bateson, M. Mother-infant exchanges: The epigenesis of conversational interaction. In D. Aronson and R. Rieber (eds.), *Developmental psycholinguistics and communicative disorders. Annals of the New York Academy of Sciences,* 263 (1975), 101–13.

Bell, S., and D. Ainsworth. Infant crying and material responsiveness. *Child Development,* 43 (1972), 1171–90.

Bellugi, U. *The acquisition of negation.* Ph.D. dissertation, Harvard University, 1967.

Berko, J. The child's learning of English morphology. *Word,* 14 (1958), 150–77.

Berko-Gleason, J. Code switching in children's language. In T. Moore (ed.), *Cognitive development and the acquisition of language.* New York: Academic Press, 1973, 159–67.

Berry, M. *Language disorders of children: The bases and diagnoses.* New York: Appleton-Century-Crofts, 1969.

Blank, M., and E. Franklin. Dialogue with preschoolers: A cognitively-based system of assessment. *Applied Psycholinguistics,* 1 (1980), 127–50.

Blank, M., M. Gessner, and A. Esposito. Language without communication: A case study. *Journal of Child Language,* 6 (1979), 329–52.

Bloom, L. *Language development: Form and function in emerging grammar.* Cambridge, Mass.: MIT Press, 1970.

Bloom, L. *One word at a time: The use of single word utterances before syntax.* The Hague: Mouton, 1973.

Bloom, L. Talking, understanding, and thinking. In R. Schiefelbusch and L. Lloyd (eds.), *Language perspectives—Acquisition, retardation, and intervention.* Baltimore: University Park Press, 1974, 285–311.

Bloom, L., and M. Lahey. *Language development and language disorders.* New York: John Wiley, 1978.

Bloom, L., P. Lightbrown, and L. Hood. Structure and variation in child language. *Monographs of the Society for Research in Child Development,* 40 (1975), 18–24.

Bloom, L., P. Miller, and L. Hood. Variation and reduction as aspects of competence in language development. In A. Pick (ed.), *Minnesota Symposia on Child Psychology.* Minneapolis: University of Minnesota Press, 9 (1975), 3–55.

Bloom, L., L. Rocissano, and L. Hood. Adult-child discourse: Developmental interaction between information processing and linguistic knowledge. *Cognitive Psychology,* 8 (1976), 521–52.

Boehm, A. *Boehm test of basic concepts.* New York: Psychological Corporation, 1971.

Bowerman, M. *Early syntactic development: A cross-linguistic study with special reference to Finnish.* London: Cambridge University Press, 1973a.

Bowerman, M. Structural relationships in children's utterances: Syntactic or semantic? In T. Moore (ed.), *Cognitive development and the acquisition of language.* New York: Academic Press, 1973b, 197–213.

Bowerman, M. Discussion summary: Development of concepts underlying language. In R. Schiefelbusch and L. Lloyd (eds.), *Language perspectives—Acquisition, retardation, and intervention.* Baltimore: University Park Press, 1974, 191–209.

Bowerman, M. Semantic factors in the acquisition of rules for word use and sentence construction. In D. Morehead and A. Morehead (eds.), *Normal and deficient child language.* Baltimore: University Park Press, 1976, 99–179.

Bowerman, M. Semantic and syntactic development: A review of what, when, and how in language acquisition. In R. Schiefelbusch (ed.), *Bases of language intervention.* Baltimore: University Park Press, 1978a, 97–189.

Bowerman, M. Words and sentences: Uniformity, individual variation, and shifts over time in patterns of acquisition. In F. Minifie and L. Lloyd (eds.), *Communicative and cognitive abilities—Early behavioral assessment.* Baltimore: University Park Press, 1978b, 349–96.

Bradley, D. Parameters of communication with infants and young children. *Allied Health and Behavioral Sciences,* 1 (1978), 550–566.

Braine, M. Children's first word combinations. *Monographs of the Society for Research in Child Development,* 41 (1976).

Brown, R. *Words and things.* Glencoe, Ill.: Free Press, 1958.

Brown, R. Language and categories. In J. Bruner, J. Goodnow, and G. Austin, *A study of thinking.* New York: John Wiley, 1967, 247–312.

Brown, R. The development of wh-questions in child speech. *Journal of Verbal Learning and Verbal Behavior,* 7 (1968), 279–90.

References

Brown, R. *A first language: The early stages.* Cambridge, Mass.: Harvard University Press, 1973.

Brown, R., and U. Bellugi. Three processes in the child's acquisition of syntax. *Harvard Educational Review,* 34 (1964), 133–51.

Brown, R., and C. Fraser. The acquisition of syntax. *Monographs of the Society for Research in Child Development,* 29 (1964), 43–79.

Brown, R., and C. Hanlon. Derivational complexity and order of acquisition in child speech. In J. Hayes (ed.), *Cognition and the development of language.* New York: John Wiley, 1970, 155–207.

Bruner, J. The ontogenesis of speech acts. *Journal of Child Language,* 2 (1975), 1–19.

Bruner, J. From communication to language: A psychological perspective. In I. Markova (ed.), *The social context of language.* New York: John Wiley, 1978, 17–48.

Carrow, E. *Test of auditory comprehension of language.* Austin, Tex: Learning Concepts, 1973.

Carrow, E. *Elicited language inventory.* Austin, Tex.: Learning Concepts, 1974.

Chafe, W. *Meaning and the structure of language.* Chicago: University of Chicago Press, 1970.

Chapman, R. Exploring children's communicative intents. In J. Miller, *Assessing language production in children.* Baltimore: University Park Press, 1981, 111–36.

Charney, R. The comprehension of "here" and "there." *Journal of Child Language,* 6 (1979), 69–80.

Chomsky, N. *Syntactic structures.* The Hague: Mouton, 1957.

Chomsky, N. *Aspects of the theory of syntax.* Cambridge, Mass.: MIT Press, 1965.

Clancy, P., T. Jacobsen, and M. Silva. The acquisition of conjunction: A cross-linguistic study. Stanford University Committee on Linguistics, *Papers and reports in child language development,* (1976), 71–80.

Clark, E. What's in a word? On the child's acquisition of semantics in his first language. In T. Moore (ed.), *Cognitive development and the acquisition of language.* New York: Academic Press, 1973, 65–110.

Clark, E. Some aspects of the conceptual basis for first language acquisition. In R. Schiefelbusch and L. Lloyd (eds.), *Language Perspectives—Acquisition, Retardation, and Intervention.* Baltimore: University Park Press, 1974, 105–28.

Clark, E. Strategies and the mapping problem in first language acquisition. In J. Macnamara (ed.), *Language learning and thought.* New York: Academic Press, 1977, 147–68.

Clark, E., and O. Garnica. Is he coming or going? On the acquisition of deictic verbs. *Journal of Verbal Learning and Verbal Behavior,* 13 (1974), 559–72.

Clark, E., and C. Sengul. Strategies in the acquisition of deixis. *Journal of Child Language,* 5 (1978), 457–75.

Clark, H., and S. Haviland. Comprehension and the given-new contract. In R. Freedle (ed.), *Discourse production and comprehension, Vol. 1.* Norwood, N.J.: Ablex Publishing Corporation, 1977, 1–40.

Cole, P. *The influence of certain semantic factors on syntax of normal and language disordered children.* Ph.D. dissertation, University of Texas, 1976.

Curtiss, S., C. Prutting, and E. Lowell. Pragmatic and semantic development in young children with impaired hearing. *Journal of Speech and Hearing Research,* 22 (1979), 534–52.

Dale, P. Is early pragmatic development measurable? *Journal of Child Language,* 7 (1980), 1–12.

Dever, R. A comparison of the results of a revised version of Berko's test of morphology with free speech of mentally retarded children. *Journal of Speech and Hearing Research,* 15 (1972), 169–78.

de Villiers, J., and P. de Villiers. A cross-sectional study of the acquisition of grammatical morphemes. *Journal of Psycholinguistic Research,* 2 (1973), 267–78.

de Villiers, J., and P. de Villiers. *Language acquisition.* Cambridge, Mass.: Harvard University Press, 1978.

Dore, J. A pragmatic description of early language development. *Journal of Psycholinguistic Research,* 3 (1974), 343–50.

Dore, J. Holophrases, speech acts and language universals. *Journal of Child Language,* 2 (1975), 21–40.

Dore, J. Children's illocutionary acts. In R. Freedle (ed.), *Discourse production and comprehension, Vol. 1.* Norwood, N.J.: Ablex Publishing Corporation, 1977, 227–44.

Dore, J. Conditions for the acquisition of speech acts. In I. Markova (ed.), *The social context of language.* New York: John Wiley, 1978, 87–112.

Dore, J., M. Gearhart, and D. Newman. The structure of nursery school conversation. In K. Nelson (ed.), *Children's language,* Vol. I. New York: Gardner Press, 1978, 337–95.

Dunn, L. *Peabody Picture Vocabulary Test.* Circle Pines, Minn: American Guidance Service, 1965.

Edinberg, G., N. Zinberg, and W. Kelman. *Clinical interviewing and counseling: Principles and techniques.* New York: Appleton-Century-Crofts, 1975.

Ervin-Tripp, S. Discourse agreement: How children answer questions. In J. Hayes (ed.), *Cognition and the development of language.* New York: John Wiley, 1970.

Fay, W., and A. Schuler. *Emerging language in autistic children.* Baltimore: University Park Press, 1980.

Fey, M., L. Leonard, and K. Wilcox. Speech style modifications of language disordered children. *Proceedings from the first Wisconsin symposium on research in child language disorders.* Madison, Wis.: University Book Store, 1980, 239–49.

Fillmore, C. The case for case. In E. Bach and R. Harms (eds.), *Universals in linguistic theory.* New York: Holt, Rinehart & Winston, 1968, 1–88.

Freedman, P., and R. Carpenter. Semantic relations used by normal and language-impaired children at stage 1. *Journal of Speech and Hearing Research,* 19 (1976), 784–95.

Gallagher, T. Contingent query sequences within adult-child discourse. *Journal of Child Language,* 8 (1981), 51–62.

Garnica, O. Some prosodic and paralinguistic features of speech to young children. In C. Snow and C. Ferguson (eds.), *Talking to children: Language input and acquisition.* New York: Cambridge University Press, 1978, 63–88.

Garvey, C. Requests and responses in children's speech. *Journal of Child Language,* 2 (1975), 41–63.

Garvey, C. The contingent query: A dependent act in conversation. In M. Lewis and L. Rosenblum (eds.), *Interaction, conversation, and the development of language.* New York: John Wiley, 1977, 63–94.

Geller, E., and S. Wollner. A preliminary investigation of the communicative competence of three linguistically impaired children. Paper presented at the New York State Speech and Hearing Association, 1976, at Grossingers.

Ginsburg, H., and S. Opper. *Piaget's theory of intellectual development,* 2nd ed. Englewood Cliffs, N.J.: Prentice Hall, 1979.

Gorth, W., and R. Hambleton. Measurement considerations for criterion-referenced testing and special education. *Journal of Special Education,* 6 (1972), 303–14.

Greenfield, P., and J. Smith. *The structure of communication in early language development.* New York: Academic Press, 1976.

Grice, H. Logic and conversation. In P. Cole and J. Morgan (eds.), *Syntax and semantics, Vol. 3: Speech Acts.* New York: Academic Press, 1975.

Halliday, M. A. K. *Explorations in the functions of language.* New York: Elsevier North-Holland, 1973.

Halliday, M. A. K. *Learning how to mean: Explorations in the development of language.* New York: Elsevier North-Holland, 1977.

Holland, A. Language therapy for children: Some thoughts on context and content. *Journal of Speech and Hearing Disorders,* 40 (1975), 514–23.

Horgan, D. How to answer questions when you've got nothing to say. *Journal of Child Language,* 4 (1977), 159–65.

Huttenlocher, J. The origins of language comprehension. In R. Solso (ed.), *Theories in cognitive psychology.* Potomac, Md.: Lawrence Erlbaum Associates, 1974.

Ingram, D. If and when transformations are acquired by children. In D. Dato (ed.), *Georgetown University Round Table on Language and Linguistics.* Washington, D.C.: Georgetown University Press, 1975, 99–127.

Johnston, J., and T. Schery. The use of grammatical morphemes by children with communication disorders. In D. Morehead and A. Morehead (eds.), *Normal and deficient child language.* Baltimore: University Park Press, 1976, 239–58.

Keenan, E. Conversational competence in children. *Journal of Child Language,* 1 (1974), 163–83.

Kirk, S., J. McCarthy, and W. Kirk. *The Illinois Test of Psycholinguistic Abilities.* Urbana, Ill.: University of Illinois Press, 1968.

Klee, T., and R. Paul. A comparison of six structural analysis procedures: A case study. In J. Miller (ed.), *Assessing language production in children.* Baltimore: University Park Press, 1981, 73–110.

Lahey, M., and L. Bloom. Planning a first lexicon: Which words to teach first. *Journal of Speech and Hearing Disorders,* 42 (1977), 340–50.

Lee, L. *Developmental Sentence Analysis.* Evanston, Ill.: Northwestern University Press, 1974.

Leonard, L. What is deviant language? *Journal of Speech and Hearing Disorders,* 37 (1972), 427–46.

Leonard, L. *Meaning in child language.* New York: Grune and Stratton, 1976.

Leonard, L., J. Bolders, and J. Miller. An examination of the semantic relations reflected in the language usage of normal and language-disordered children. *Journal of Speech and Hearing Research,* 19 (1976), 371–92.

Lewis, M. The infant and its caregiver: The role of contingency. *Allied Health and Behavioral Sciences,* 1 (1978), 469–92.

Lewis, M., and S. Goldberg. Perceptual-cognitive development in infancy: A generalized expectancy model as a function of the mother-child interaction. *Merrill-Palmer Quarterly,* 15 (1969), 81–100.

Limber, J. The genesis of complex sentences. In T. Moore (ed.), *Cognitive development and the acquisition of language.* New York: Academic Press, 1973, 169–85.

Longhurst, T., and S. Grubb. A comparison of language samples collected in four situations. *Language, Speech, and Hearing Services in the Schools,* 5 (1974), 71–78.

McCarthy, D. McCarthy scales of children's abilities. New York: Psychological Corporation, 1974.

McDonald, E. *Understanding those feelings.* Pittsburgh: Stanwix House, 1962.

MacDonald, J., and J. Blott. Environmental language intervention: The rationale for a diagnostic and training strategy through rules, context, and generalization. *Journal of Speech and Hearing Disorders,* 39 (1974), 244–56.

MacDonald, J., and M. Nickols. *The environmental language inventory.* Columbus, Ohio: Nisonger Center, Ohio State University, 1974.

McNeill, D. The creation of language by children. In J. Lyons and R. Wales (eds.), *Psycholinguistic papers.* Edinburgh: Edinburgh University Press, 1966a, 99–115.

McNeill, D. Developmental psycholinguistics. In F. Smith and G. Miller (eds.), *The genesis of language: A psycholinguistic approach.* Cambridge, Mass.: MIT Press, 1966b.

McNeill, D. *The acquisition of language: The study of developmental psycholinguistics.* New York: Harper & Row, Pub., 1970.

Maratsos, M. Nonegocentric communicative abilities in preschool children. *Child Development,* 44 (1973), 697–700.

Menyuk, P. Comparison of grammar of children with functionally deviant and normal speech. *Journal of Speech and Hearing Research,* 7 (1964), 109–21.

Menyuk, P. *Sentences children use.* Cambridge, Mass.: MIT Press, 1969.

Miller, J. Assessing children's language behavior: A developmental process approach. In R. Schiefelbusch (ed.), *Bases of language intervention,* 1978, 269–318.

Miller, J. *Assessing language production in children: Experimental procedures.* Baltimore: University Park Press, 1981.

Miller, J., and D. Yoder. An ontogenetic language teaching strategy for retarded children. In R. Schiefelbusch and L. Lloyd (eds.), *Language perspectives—Acquisition, retardation, and intervention.* Baltimore: University Park Press, 1974, 505–28.

References

Miller, L. Pragmatics and early childhood language disorders: Communicative interactions in a half-hour sample. *Journal of Speech and Hearing Disorders,* 3 (1978), 419–36.

Moerk, E. Verbal interactions between children and their mothers during the preschool years. *Journal of Developmental Psychology,* 11 (1975), 788–94.

Morehead, D., and D. Ingram. The development of base syntax in normal and linguistically deviant children. *Journal of Speech and Hearing Research,* 16 (1973), 330–52.

Morehead, D., and A. Morehead. From signal to sign: A Piagetian view of thought and language during the first two years. In R. Schiefelbusch and L. Lloyd (eds.), *Language perspectives—Acquisition, retardation, and intervention.* Baltimore: University Park Press, 1974, 153–90.

Musselwhite, C., K. St. Louis, and P. Penick. A communicative interaction analysis system for language disordered children. *Journal of Communication Disorders,* 13 (1980), 315–24.

Nelson, K. Structure and strategy in learning to talk. *Monographs of the Society for Research in Child Development,* 38 (1973).

Nelson, K. Concept, word and sentence: Interrelations in acquisition and development. *Psychological Review,* 81 (1974), 267–85.

Nelson, K. Some attributes of adjectives used by young children. *Cognition,* 4 (1976), 13–30.

Nelson, K. The conceptual basis for naming. In J. Macnamara (ed.), *Language learning and thought.* New York: Academic Press, 1977, 117–36.

Nelson, L., and M. Weber-Olsen. The elicited language inventory and the influence of contextual cues. *Journal of Speech and Hearing Disorders,* 45 (1980), 549–63.

Piaget, J., and B. Inhelder. *The psychology of the child.* New York: Basic Books, 1969.

Pick, A. Perception in the acquisition of reading. In F. Murray and J. Pikulski (eds.), *The acquisition of reading: Cognitive, linguistic, and perceptual prerequisites.* Baltimore: University Park Press, 1978, 99–122.

Porch, B. *Porch index of communicative ability in children.* Palo Alto, Calif.: Consulting Psychologist Press, 1974.

Prutting, C. Process: The action of moving forward progressively from one point to another on the way to completion. *Journal of Speech and Hearing Disorders,* 44 (1979), 3–30.

Prutting, C., N. Bagshaw, H. Goldstein, S. Juskowitz, and I. Umen. Clinician-child discourse: Some preliminary questions. *Journal of Speech and Hearing Disorders,* 43 (1978), 123–39.

Prutting, C., T. Gallagher, and A. Mulac. The expressive portion of the NSST compared to a spontaneous language sample. *Journal of Speech and Hearing Disorders,* 40 (1975), 40–48.

Pylyshyn, Z. What does it take to bootstrap a language? In J. Macnamara (ed.), *Language learning and thought.* New York: Academic Press, 1977, 37–45.

Rees, N. Noncommunicative functions of language in children. *Journal of Speech and Hearing Disorders,* 38 (1973), 98–110.

Rees, N. Pragmatics of language: Applications to normal and disordered language development. In R. Schiefelbusch (ed.), *Bases of language intervention.* Baltimore: University Park Press, 1978, 191–268.

Richardson, S. Myth-Communication. In A. Simmons-Martin and D. Calvert (eds.), *Parent-infant intervention: Communication disorders.* New York: Grune and Stratton, 1979, 73–87.

Rodgon, M. Knowing what to say and wanting to say it: Some communicative and structural aspects of single-word responses to questions. *Journal of Child Language,* 6 (1979), 81–90.

Rodgon, M., W. Jankowski, and L. Alenskas. A multi-functional approach to single-word usage. *Journal of Child Language,* 4 (1977), 23–43.

Rom, A., and L. Bliss. A comparison of verbal communicative skills of language impaired and normal speaking children. *Journal of Communication Disorders,* 14 (1981), 133–40.

Sachs, J. The adaptive significance of linguistic input to prelinguistic infants. In C. Snow and C. Ferguson (eds.), *Talking to children: Language input and acquisition.* New York: Cambridge University Press, 1978, 51–61.

Schery, T. Selecting assessment strategies for language-disordered children. *Topics in Language Disorders,* 1 (1981), 59–73.

Schlesinger, I. Production of utterances and language acquisition. In D. Slobin (ed.), *The ontogenesis of grammar.* New York: Academic Press, 1971, 63–101.

Schlesinger, I. Relational concepts underlying language. In R. Schiefelbusch and L. Lloyd (eds.), *Language perspectives—Acquisition, retardation, and intervention.* Baltimore: University Park Press, 1974, 129–51.

Scott, K. The rationale and methodological considerations underlying early cognitive and behavioral assessment. In F. Minifie and L. Lloyd (eds.), *Communicative and cognitive abilities—Early behavioral assessment.* Baltimore: University Park Press, 1978, 3–20.

Searle, J. *Speech acts: An essay in the philosophy of language.* London: Cambridge University Press, 1969.

Shatz, M., and R. Gelman. Beyond syntax: The influence of conversational constraints on speech modification. In C. Snow and C. Ferguson (eds.), *Talking to children, Language input and acquisition.* New York: Cambridge University Press, 1978, 189–98.

Siegel, G., and P. Broen. Language assessment. In L. Lloyd (ed.), *Communication assessment and intervention strategies.* Baltimore: University Park Press, 1976, 73–122.

Siegel, G., and J. Spradlin. Programming for language and communication therapy. In R. Schiefelbusch (ed.), *Language intervention strategies.* Baltimore: University Park Press, 1978, 357–98.

Simon, C. *Communicative competence: Pragmatic approach to language therapy.* Tucson, Ariz.: Communication Skill Builders, Inc., 1980.

Sinclair, H. Developmental psycholinguistics. In D. Elkind and J. Flavell (eds.), *Studies in cognitive development.* New York: Oxford University Press, 1969, 315–36.

Sinclair, H. Sensorimotor action patterns as a condition for the acquisition of syntax. In R. Huxley and E. Ingram (eds.), *Language acquisition: Models and methods.* New York: Academic Press, 1971.

Sinclair-de Swart, H. Language acquisition and cognitive development. In T. Moore (ed.), *Cognitive development and the acquisition of language.* New York: Academic Press, 1973, 9–25.

Slobin, D. Cognitive prerequisites for the development of grammar. In C. Ferguson and D. Slobin (eds.), *Studies of child language development.* New York: Holt, Rinehart & Winston, 1973.

Snow, C. The development of conversation between mothers and babies. *Journal of Child Language,* 4 (1977), 1–22.

Snow, C. Mother's speech research: From input to interaction. In C. Snow and C. Ferguson (eds.), *Talking to children: Language input and acquisition.* New York: Cambridge University Press, 1978, 31–49.

Snyder, L. *Pragmatics in language disabled children: Their prelinguistic and early verbal performatives and presuppositions.* Ph.D. dissertation, University of Colorado, Denver, 1975.

Snyder, L. Communicative and cognitive abilities and disabilities in the sensorimotor period. *Merrill Palmer Quarterly,* 24 (1978), 161–80.

Snyder, L. Assessing communicative abilities in the sensorimotor period: Content and context. *Topics in Language Disorders,* 1 (1981), 31–46.

Stark, R. Infant speech production and communication skills. *Allied Health and Behavioral Sciences,* 1 (1978), 131–51.

Stern, D. *The first relationship: Infant and Mother.* Cambridge, Mass.: Harvard University Press, 1977.

Stern, D., J. Jaffe, B. Beebe, and S. Bennett. Vocalizing in unison and in alteration: Two modes of communication within the mother-infant dyad. In L. Bloom (ed.), *Readings in language development.* New York: John Wiley, 1978, 115–27.

Stremel, K., and C. Waryas. A behavioral-psycholinguistic approach to language training. In L. McReynolds (ed.), *Developing systematic procedures for training children's language. Asha Monograph,* 18. Danville, Ill.: Interstate Press, 1974.

Templin, M. Certain language skills in children: Their development and interrelationships. *Child Welfare Monograph No. 26.* Minneapolis: University of Minnesota Press, 1957.

Terman, L., and M. Merrill. *Stanford-Binet Intelligence Scale.* Boston: Houghton Mifflin Co., 1960.

Tjossem, T. (ed.). *Intervention strategies for high risk infants and young children.* Baltimore: University Park Press, 1976.

Tyack, D., and R. Gottsleben. *Language sampling, analysis, and training: A handbook for teachers and clinicians.* Palo Alto, Calif.: Consulting Psychologist Press, 1974.

Umiker-Sebeok, D. Preschool children's interconversational narratives. *Journal of Child Language,* 6 (1979), 91–109.

Uzgiris, I., and J. Hunt. *Assessment in infancy.* Urbana, Ill.: University of Illinois Press, 1975.

Wales, R., and R. Campbell. The development of comparison and the comparison of development. In G. Flores d'Arcais and W. Levelt (eds.), *Advances in psycholinguistics.* Amsterdam: North-Holland Publishing Company, 1970.

Waryas, C., and K. Stremel-Campbell. Grammatical training for the language-delayed child: A new perspective. In R. Schiefelbusch (ed.), *Language intervention strategies.* Baltimore: University Park Press, 1978, 145–92.

Wells, G. Learning to code experience through language. *Journal of Child Language,* 1 (1974), 243–69.

Wood, M. *An analysis of selected morphemes in the spontaneous speech of normal and language-impaired children.* Ph.D. dissertation, University of Texas, Austin, 1976.

INDEX

Actions. *See also* Semantic roles
  alternate actions, 13, 14, 17, 48, 109-10, 113-14
  coactions, 12, 13, 16, 17, 34, 108-9
  reciprocal actions, 15, 17, 48, 113-14
Ainsworth, D., 15
Alenskas, L, 95
Anglin, J., 53, 55, 57, 59
Aram, D., 4
Assessment, 86-98. *See also* Language samples
  of content, 89, 95-96, 97
  criterion-referenced procedures, 86, 94
  of form, 89, 96, 97, 98
  nonstandardized procedures, 86, 94
  norm-referenced procedures, 86, 94
  observation process, 87, 91-93
  parent participation, 87-91, 92
  of prelinguistic development, 86
  purpose, 86, 87
  standardized procedures, 86, 93, 97, 98
  of use 88-89, 92-93, 94-95, 97
Attention directing, 12, 14, 15, 16, 17, 21, 47, 48, 107, 108
Attention sharing, 12, 14, 17, 107, 108, 109, 111
Ausberger, C., 163
Austin, J., 20

Bagshaw, N., 95
Baltaxe, C., 49
Bangs, T., 4, 90
Bates, E., 14, 16, 18, 21, 40, 42, 43
Bateson, M., 34
Beebe, B., 12, 13, 14
Bell, S., 15
Bellugi, U., 71, 80
Bennett, S., 12, 13, 14
Berko, J., 43, 97
Berry, M., 90
Blank, M., 30, 95
Bliss, L., 30
Bloom, L., 5, 6, 14, 21, 33, 34, 35, 43, 51, 52, 55, 57, 62, 63, 65, 69, 70, 71, 73, 74, 80, 82, 86, 94, 95, 97, 147
Blott, J., 96, 163
Boehm, A., 97
Bolders, J., 67, 96
Bowerman, M., 3, 6, 55, 57, 58, 63, 65, 69, 71
Bradley, D., 15
Braine, M., 71

Broen, P., 86
Brown, R., 3, 6, 21, 41, 42, 47, 48, 52, 56, 59, 62, 63, 64, 65, 66, 68, 69, 71, 73, 74, 75, 76, 77, 79, 80, 81, 83, 84, 91, 96
Bruner, J., 6, 11, 12, 13, 14, 15, 21, 34, 47, 107

Camaioni, L., 21
Campbell, R., 58
Caregiver-child interactions. *See also* Attention directing; Attention sharing; Interaction routines
  models for language use, 10-13, 15, 34, 47, 109
  parental responsiveness, 14, 15, 56
  and social/affective development, 12, 13, 15, 17, 108, 109
Carpenter, R., 67
Carrow, E., 97, 98
Chafe, W., 53, 61, 64
Chapman, R., 95
Charney, R., 47
Chomsky, N., 69
Clancy, P., 96
Clark, E., 46, 47, 48, 52, 58, 59
Clark, H., 39
Cole, P., 85
Compositional meanings. *See* Propositions
Content of language. *See* Semantics; Referential meanings; Propositions
Context of language. *See also* Presuppositions
  and code switching, 43
  and language content, 40-48
  and selecting form, 14, 40-46
Conversational acts. *See* Functions of utterances
Conversational Exchanges. *See also* Deixis
  clarifying meaning, 33, 136-38
  gaining listeners' attention, 34, 36, 37, 121, 128
  grammatical ellipsis, 33, 34, 35, 129
  linguistic contingency, 33, 34-36, 38, 129
  prelinguistic routines, 12-13, 15, 17, 108-10, 114
  pronominalization, 33, 34, 35
  regulating exchanges, 24, 29, 109-10, 113, 128
  topic maintenance, 33, 34, 37, 38, 129
  turn-taking, 33, 34, 37, 109-10, 114, 128

175

Conversational implicatures, 33
Cooperative principles, 32-33
Copular structures, 72, 73, 74
Covocalizations. *See* Coactions
Curtiss, S., 29, 30

Dale, P., 94, 95, 97
Declaratives, 16, 30, 68, 79, 80, 81
Deixis, 15, 46-51, 138-46
    of person, 14, 46, 47, 48-49, 139-41
    of place, 14, 46, 48, 50, 141-43
    of time, 46, 47, 50, 143-46
Demand mode of behavior, 14, 15, 107, 110-13
Dever, R., 91
de Villiers, J., 42, 43, 47, 54, 55, 56, 57, 58, 59, 69, 83
de Villiers, P., 42, 43, 47, 54, 55, 56, 57, 58, 59, 69, 83
Dialogue. *See* Conversational exchanges
Dore, J., 6, 16, 19, 22, 25, 28, 29, 31, 32, 62, 94
Dunn, L., 97

Edinburg, G., 87
Ervin-Tripp, S., 82
Esposito, A., 30
Exchange mode of behavior, 15, 107, 113-14
Expansions of utterances:
    coordination, 79
    embedding, 79
    number of semantic relations, 65-66, 67, 71-74, 150-54, 156

Fay, W., 49
Fey, M., 46, 91
Fillmore, C., 61, 64
Form of language. *See also* Expansions of utterances; Grammatical morphemes; Prepositions; Sentence forms; Syntax
    and meaning, 38, 155-59
    and pragmatic intent, 40, 68, 154-55
    and social environment, 40-41, 42, 43, 45
Franklin, E., 95
Fraser, C., 71
Freedman, P., 67
Functions of language. *See also* Speech acts
    communicative, 2-4, 18, 21, 22
    heuristic, 23, 111, 112, 125-27
    ideational, 23, 24-25, 32, 125-27
    imaginative, 15, 23
    informative, 23, 24, 31, 123-24
    instrumental, 22, 23, 31, 80, 111, 115-19
    interactional, 13, 22, 23, 31, 111, 112, 119-23
    interpersonal, 23, 24, 25, 32, 115-24
    mathetic, 23, 24, 25, 31, 32, 125-27, 152
    multifunctions, 24, 25, 127
    noncommunicative, 2, 4, 18
    personal, 23, 111, 112, 135
    pragmatic, 23, 24, 25, 31, 115-24, 152
    regulatory, 22, 23, 31, 80, 111, 119-21
    textual, 23, 25
Functions of utterances:
    assertives, 25, 26, 27, 32
    expressives, 25, 26, 27, 29, 31, 32
    performatives, 25, 26, 27, 28, 31, 32
    regulatives, 25, 26, 29, 31, 32
    requestives, 25, 26, 27, 31, 32
    responsives, 25, 26, 27, 28, 32

Gallagher, T., 91, 95
Garnica, O., 48
Garvey, C., 44, 80, 95
Gearhart, M., 22, 25, 28, 29, 31, 32
Geller, E., 30
Gelman, R., 43, 44
Gessner, M., 30
Ginsberg, H., 12, 13, 15
Goldberg, S., 12
Goldstein, H., 95
Gorth, W., 94
Gottsleben, R., 96
Grammatical morphemes, 68, 75-79, 157-59
    articles, 76, 77, 78
    contractible auxiliary, 76, 77, 79
    contractible copula, 76, 77, 78
    in and *on* (*see also* Deixis of place), 74, 76, 77, 78
    irregular past tense (*see also* Deixis of time), 76, 77, 78
    plural markers, 75, 76, 77, 78
    possessive markers (*see also* Deixis of person), 76, 77, 78
    present progressive, 75, 76, 77
    regular past tense (*see also* Deixis of time), 75, 76, 77, 78
    third person irregular, 76, 77, 78
    third person regular, 76, 77, 78
    uncontractible auxiliary, 76, 77, 79
Greenfield, P., 20, 21, 41, 42, 58, 62, 94
Grice, H., 32, 33
Grubb, S., 91

Halliday, M.A.K., 2, 3, 6, 21, 22, 23, 24, 25, 29, 31, 32, 94, 125
Hambleton, R., 94
Hanlon, C., 81
Haviland, S., 39
Holland, A., 7, 147
Hood, L., 34, 35, 55, 65, 71, 73, 74, 80
Horgan, D., 81
Hunt, J., 86
Huttenlocher, J., 55

Imperatives, 16, 30, 68, 80-81
Ingram, D., 69, 84
Inhelder, B., 6, 15
Intentional acts. *See also* Functions of language; functions of utterances
    encoding intentions, 17, 18-32, 114-27
    prelinguistic acts, 10, 15, 16, 17, 21, 30, 110-13
Interaction mode of behavior, 12, 107, 108-9

Interaction routines, 11, 12, 13, 17, 33, 34, 36, 37, 109-10, 113-14, 122. *See also* Actions; conversational exchanges
Intervention:
    definition, 7
    for disorders of content, 146-54
    for disorders of form, 154-61
    for disorders of use, 114-46
    need for, 2-4
    for prelinguistic disorders, 106-14
    purposes, 4, 101, 102, 103
    setting, 4, 101-5

Jacobson, T., 96
Jaffe, J., 12, 13, 14
Jankowski, W., 95
Johnston, J., 84
Juskowitz, S., 95

Keenan, E., 34
Kelman, W., 87
Kirk, S., 97
Kirk, W., 97
Klee, T., 97

Lahey, M., 5, 6, 14, 33, 34, 35, 43, 51, 52, 63, 65, 70, 73, 82, 86, 94, 95, 97, 147
Language samples. *See also* Assessment
    analysis, 94-97
    obtaining, 91-93
    recording, 93-94
Lee, L., 91, 96, 163
Leonard, L., 46, 63, 65, 67, 69, 74, 84, 91, 96
Lewis, M., 6, 12, 107
Lexical development. *See* Referential meanings
Lightbrown, P., 55, 65, 73
Limber, J., 82, 83, 84
Line of regard. *See* Attention sharing
Longhurst, T., 91
Lowell, E., 29, 30

McCarthy, D., 97
McCarthy, J., 97
McDonald, E., 87
MacDonald, J., 96, 97, 163
McNeill, D., 69
Maratsos, M., 43
Menyuk, P., 69, 84, 85
Merrill, M., 97
Miller, J., 67, 86, 87, 91, 93, 94, 95, 96, 97, 163
Miller, L., 163
Miller, P., 35, 71, 74, 80
Moerk, E., 95
Morehead, A., 13
Morehead, D., 13, 69, 84
Morphology. *See* Grammatical morphemes
Mulac, A., 91
Musselwhite, C., 95

Nation, J., 4
Nelson, K., 3, 24, 55, 56
New information. *See* Presuppositions
Newman, D., 22, 25, 28, 29, 31, 32
Nickols, M., 97

Old information. *See* Presuppositions
Operations of reference:
    denial, 63, 69, 80, 150-53
    nomination, 63, 150-52
    nonexistence, 63, 69, 79, 150-52
    recurrence, 63, 69, 80, 150-52
    rejection, 21, 63, 69, 80, 150-52
Opper, S., 12, 13, 15

Paul, R., 97
Penick, P., 95
Performatives, 20, 21, 28, 30, 60, 114
Piaget, J., 6, 15
Pick, A., 4
Porch, B., 97
Pragmatics, 6, 11, 15, 18, 68-69, 114-46. *See also,* Caregiver-child interactions; Conversational exchanges; Deixis; Functions of language; Functions of utterances; Intentional acts; Interaction routines; Presuppositions; Speech acts
Precursors to language, 11-16, 36, 106-14
Preintentional acts, 10, 12-15, 16-18, 21, 108, 109, 110, 111
Prepositions, 69, 70, 74-75, 156-57. *See also* Grammatical morphemes
Presuppositions, 38-46, 130-36
    knowledge of the world, 40, 132-34
    linguistic context, 39, 44, 131-32
    new-old information, 39-44, 130-34
    nonlinguistic context, 39, 42, 44, 130-31
    social/cultural expectations, 40-41, 43-45, 134-36
Propositions, 11, 16, 19, 21, 22, 29, 36, 51, 52, 61-68, 95, 150-54
Protodeclaratives, 16
Protoimperatives, 16
Prutting, C., 29, 30, 91, 94, 95
Pylyshyn, Z., 21

Questions. *See* Sentence forms

Rees, N., 4, 15, 18, 25, 30, 46
Reference shifting, 46, 47, 48, 50, 54, 58. *See also* Deixis
Referential meanings, 11, 16, 21, 24, 36, 51, 52-61, 95, 146, 147-50
    adult imput, 55, 56, 57
    hierarchical relationships, 53, 54, 59, 60
    overextensions, 57-58, 60
    semantic features, 52, 56, 58
    underextensions, 57-58, 60
Requests:
    direct, 40, 43-44, 81, 116-21, 135, 159, 132-34

177

Requests (*cont.*)
    indirect, 40, 43-44, 80-81, 122-23, 134, 135-36, 159
Response expectancy, 14, 15, 17, 34, 110
Richardson, S., 4
Rocissano, L., 34, 35
Rodgon, M., 35, 81, 95
Role reversals, 15, 24, 46-51, 113-14. *See also* Reference shifting
Rom, A., 30

Sachs, J., 12
St. Louis, K., 95
Schery, T., 84, 87
Schlesinger, I., 3, 69, 71
Schuler, A., 49
Scott, K., 86, 94
Searle, J., 19
Semantics, 6, 11, 51-68, 146-54. *See also* Operations of reference; Propositions; Referential meanings
    semantic relations, 61-68, 69-75, 95-96, 150-54, 155
    semantic roles:
        action, 13, 15, 64, 65, 67, 71, 72, 73, 74
        agent, 13, 15, 64, 65, 67, 71, 72, 74
        attribute, 58, 64, 65, 72-73
        beneficiary, 64, 65, 70, 72, 75
        comitative, 64, 65, 70, 74, 75
        demonstrative, 64
        entity, 64, 72-73, 74
        experiencer, 64, 65, 74
        instrument, 64, 65, 72, 74, 75
        location, 13, 64, 65, 70, 71, 72, 73, 74
        object, 64, 65, 67, 71, 74
        possession, 64, 65, 72
        possessor, 64, 65, 72
        prelinguistic forerunners, 13, 61
Sengul, C., 46, 47
Sentence forms, 79-84, 159-61
    complex:
        coordination, 79, 82-83, 160, 161
        embedding, 79, 83-84, 160, 161
    declarative, 16, 68, 79, 80, 81
    imperative, 16, 68, 79, 80-81, 159, 160
    negation, 68-69, 79-80, 159
    and pragmatic intent, 69, 79, 80, 81, 159. *See also* Requests
    question forms:
        yes/no, 35, 79, 81, 159, 161
        wh-questions, 35, 79, 81, 159, 160
        tag questions, 81
    and semantic structure, 69, 79, 80, 81, 82, 83, 159. *See also* Word order; Propositions
Shatz, M., 43, 44
Siegel, G., 7, 86
Silva, M., 96
Simmons, J., 49
Simon, C., 163

Sinclair, H., 63
Sinclair-de Swart, H., 3
Single word utterances:
    function, 21-22, 46, 55, 62
    successive single-word utterances, 70-71
    underlying structure, 61-63
    word selection, 41-42, 46, 55
Slobin, D., 3, 6, 71
Smith, J., 20, 21, 41, 42, 58, 62, 94
Snow, C., 6, 13, 14, 34
Snyder, L., 30, 45, 86, 97
Social context, 14, 17, 40-41, 43-46. *See also* Presuppositions
Speech acts:
    illocutionary acts (force), 14, 16, 19, 20, 21, 22, 24, 25, 94
    perlocutionary acts (force), 14, 19
    propositional acts, 19, 29
    utterance acts, 19
Spradlin, J., 7
Stark, R., 15, 107
States. *See also* Verbs
    permanent (static), 54, 55, 72, 73, 74
    transitory, 54, 55, 73, 74
Stern, D., 12, 13, 14, 34
Stremel, K., 163
Stremel-Campbell, K., 10, 163
Syntax, 6, 11, 24, 68-86, 164. *See also* Form of Language; Propositions; Sentence forms; Word order

Templin, M., 95
Terman, L., 97
Tjossem, T., 90
Tyack, D., 96

Umen, I., 95
Umiker-Sebeok, D., 36, 48
Uzgiris, I., 86

Verbs:
    action 53, 55, 60, 71
    ambient 53
    deictic 46, 48, 138
    process 53, 60
    state, 53, 54, 55, 60, 71. *See also* States
Vocabulary. *See* Referential Meanings
Volterra, V., 21

Wales, R., 58
Waryas, C., 10, 163
Wells, G., 42, 55
Wilcox, K., 46, 91
Wollner, S., 30
Wood, M., 75, 85
Word meaning. *See* Referential meanings
Word order, 69-74, 155-156. *See also* Expansions of utterances; Semantics; Syntax

Yoder, D., 163

Zinberg, N., 87

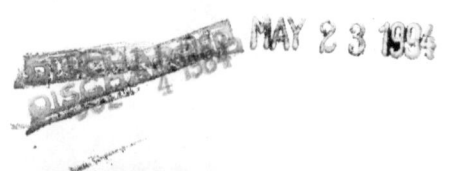